Multiple Choice Questions in
Paediatric Surgery

Multiple Choice Questions in Paediatric Surgery

A unique book of Multiple-Choice Questions in Paediatric Surgery that provides direct specific knowledge of paediatric surgery, analyse your knowledge and greatly helps in passing examination.

DR. MUHAMMAD KHALID SYED

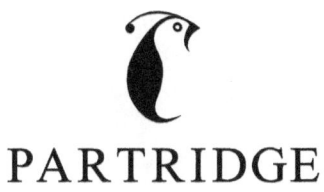

PARTRIDGE

Copyright © 2018 by Dr. Muhammad Khalid Syed.

Library of Congress Control Number:		2018949743
ISBN:	Hardcover	978-1-5437-4660-0
	Softcover	978-1-5437-4659-4
	eBook	978-1-5437-4661-7

All rights reserved. No part of this book may be used or reproduced by any means, graphic, electronic, or mechanical, including photocopying, recording, taping or by any information storage retrieval system without the written permission of the author except in the case of brief quotations embodied in critical articles and reviews.

Because of the dynamic nature of the Internet, any web addresses or links contained in this book may have changed since publication and may no longer be valid. The views expressed in this work are solely those of the author and do not necessarily reflect the views of the publisher, and the publisher hereby disclaims any responsibility for them.

Print information available on the last page.

To order additional copies of this book, contact
Toll Free 800 101 2657 (Singapore)
Toll Free 1 800 81 7340 (Malaysia)
orders.singapore@partridgepublishing.com

www.partridgepublishing.com/singapore

DEDICATION

This book is dedicated to the
Holy Prophet "MUHAMMAD" (Peace be upon him), whose teaching enlightened the world and has given a glorious vision to humanity.

Dr. Muhammad Khalid Syed

CONTENTS

Preface xiii

Section 1: Abdomen A
Pyloric Stenosis..1
Duodenal Atresia 3
Jejunal Atresia/Ileal Atresia...5
Meconeum Ileus...5
Malrotation..9
Achalasia Cardia 12
Intussusception 13
Vitellointestinal Duct Anomalies.................................... 15
Omphalocele and Gastroschisis 19
Ascites 24
Trichobezoar 25

Section 2: Abdomen B
Pancreas 26
Portal Hypertension 29
Biliary Atresia..30
Choledochal Cyst...34
Splenectomy 37
Hirschsprung's Disease..38

Anorectal Malformation 44
Necrotising Enterocolitis 48
Antegrade Continent Catheterizable Stoma 50
Rectal Prolapse 52
Ulcerative Colitis 53
Crohn's Disease 55

Section 3: Abdomen C
Inguinal Hernia 58
Umbilical Hernia 60
Circumcision 61
Bleeding Per Rectum 61
Short Bowel Syndrome 64
Mesenteric and Omental Cyst 66
Duplication of Gastrointestinal Tract 67
Primary Peritonitis 69
Acute Appendicitis 69
Intestinal Parasites 71
Liver Abscess 73

Section 4: Urology A
Urinary Incontinence, Enuresis, and Bladder
Reconstructive Procedures 74
Urolithiasis 78
Vesicoureteric Reflux 81
Partial Nephrectomy 84
Ureteric Duplication, Ectopic Ureter, and Ureterocele ... 84
Mega Ureter and Prune-Belly Syndrome 86

Diversion and Undiversion 88
Posterior Urethral Valve 88

Section 5: Urology B
Renal Agenesis, Dysplasia and Cystic Disease, Renal
Fusion, and Ectopia 92
Pelviureteric Junction Obstruction 93
Exstrophy Bladder 95
Hypospadias 97
Cloacal Exstrophy 99
Ambiguous Genitalia 100
Testicular Torsion 102
Undescended Testes 103

Section 6: Thoracic Surgery
Congenital Diaphragmatic Hernia 106
Oesophageal Atresia 111
Aortopexy 117
Oesophageal Replacement 117
Caustic Ingestion 118
Gastroesophageal Reflux 120
Thoracic Cavity 123
Chest Wall 130

Section 7: Head and Neck and Soft Tissue Lesions
Head and Neck 133
Soft Tissue Lesions 139

Section 8: Orthopedic

Digital Malformation 141

Spina Bifida 142

Telipes Equinovarus 143

Developmental Dysplasia of Hip 145

Septic Arthritis 147

Osteomylitis 147

Femur Fracture 148

Ingrown Toenail 150

Section 9: Trauma

Abdominal Trauma 152

Urogenital Injury 157

Burn 159

Thoracic Trauma 163

Child Abuse 164

Birth Trauma 165

Section 10: Oncology

General Oncology 166

Central Nervous System Tumour 167

Teratoma and Germ Cell Tumour 170

Sarcoma 173

Ovarian Lesions 175

Liver Tumours 176

Wilms Tumour 178

Lymphoma 179

Pheochromocytoma 182

Neuroblastoma 184
Bone Tumour 186
Testicular Tumour 186

Section 11: Vessels and Lymphatics
Vascular Malformation 188
Lymphatic Malformation 191

Section 12: Anatomy for Paediatric Surgeons
Thorax 194
Abdomen 197
Pelvis 206
Urogenital System 210
Limbs 213
Head and Neck 215
Vertebral Column 218

Answers 221

PREFACE

In my career, observing multiple paediatric surgical examinations, I realised there is shortage of MCQ (multiple-choice question) books that provide specific, in-depth knowledge of paediatric surgery. To fulfil the needs of candidates, I decided to write a MCQ book that contains such core knowledge. Rather than write long explanations, I attempted to provide as much information as possible within the MCQs themselves.

For each question, readers are asked to select the best answer. In most questions it is asked to select the false option out of five possible choices. The purpose of this is to provide an abundance of correct information in a direct manner, leaving little need to write explanations in the answers. Some times information is repeated in the MCQ's as the MCQs are derived from different books but this provides same information from different angles.

Most of MCQs are based on knowledge acquired from the following books:

- *Pediatric Surgery*, edited by Mark Ravitch, James A. O'Neill Jr. Mosby

- *Rob & Smith's Operative Surgery: Pediatric Surgery*, by L. Spitz and A. G. Coran
- *Last's Anatomy: Regional and Applied*, by Chummy S. Sinnatamby
- *Pediatric Surgery Secrets*, by Philip L. Glick, Richard Pearl, Michael S. Irish, and Michael G. Caty

This book has been reviewed by Dr. Ahmed Abduh Ahmad Al-Faqheeh, consultant paediatric surgeon at Al-Qunfudah General Hospital, Al-Qunfudhah, Saudi Arabia; Dr. Mumtaz, consultant paediatric surgeon at King Khalid Military City Hospital, Hafr Al Batin, Saudi Arabia; and Dr. Shahid, specialist paediatric surgeon in Biljurashi, Saudi Arabia. Dr. Abdul Raouf Goraya General Surgeon, Al-Aqiq General Hospital, KSA.

This book is beneficial for:

- All paediatric surgery examinations
- General surgical examination to cover a portion of paediatric surgery
- Paediatric medicine examination to cover differential diagnosis of surgical conditions

Dr. Muhammad Khalid Syed
MBBS, FCPS, MRCS, FEBPS, FACS

SECTION 1

ABDOMEN A

Pyloric Stenosis

Q. 1
A five-week-old baby has been projectile vomiting for two weeks, is losing weight, is dehydrated with visible gastric peristalsis and has a palpable mass in epigastrium. The most likely diagnosis is:

A. Gastroesophageal reflux.
B. Pyloric stenosis.
C. Duodenal stenosis.
D. Duodenal atresia.
E. Gastric volvulus.

Q. 2
Regarding the ultrasound finding to label hypertrophied pyloric stenosis, the most correct statement is:

- A. Pyloric muscle thickness is 4 mm or more, and pyloric channel length is 16 mm or more.
- B. Pyloric muscle thickness is 2 mm or more, and pyloric channel length is 14 mm or more.
- C. Pyloric muscle thickness is 2 mm or more, and pyloric channel length is 16 mm or more.
- D. Pyloric muscle thickness is 16 mm or more, and pyloric channel length is 10 mm or more.
- E. Pyloric muscle thickness is 8 mm or more, and pyloric channel length is 12 mm or more.

Q. 3
The preferred site of incision for pyloromyotomy is:

- A. Anterosuperior surface.
- B. Posterior surface.
- C. Posterosuperior surface.
- D. Posteroinferior surface.
- E. Inferior surface.

Q. 4
The metabolic derangement in pyloric stenosis is:

- A. Hyperchloremic, hyperkalemic metabolic alkalosis.
- B. Metabolic acidosis.
- C. Hypochloremic, hypokalemic metabolic acidosis.
- D. Hypochloremic, hypokalemic metabolic alkalosis.
- E. Hypochloremic, hyperkalemic metabolic alkalosis.

Duodenal Atresia

Q. 5
One-day-old baby with bilious vomiting; examination shows Down syndrome and epigastric fullness. X-rays show double bubble sign. The most likely diagnosis is:

    A. Oesophageal atresia.
    B. Pyloric stenosis.
    C. Duodenal atresia.
    D. Jejunal atresia.
    E. Ileal atresia.

Q. 6
Type II duodenal atresia is:

    A. Simple intraluminal membrane.
    B. Intraluminal membrane with wind-soak type.
    C. Intraluminal membrane with perforation.
    D. Intraluminal membrane with annular pancreas.
    E. Blind ends of duodenum connected with a fibrous cord.

Q. 7
In duodenal atresia, which of the following is not true?

    A. Diamond duodenostomy is a good option.
    B. Kocher's manoeuvre is needed during the operation.
    C. Either one-layer or two-layer anastomosis technique can be used.
    D. If the trans-anastomotic tube is placed, the feed is started on the fourth day.

E. The outcome depends on associated condition, anastomotic leakage, intra-abdominal sepsis and wound complication.

Q. 8
In type I duodenal atresia, the preferred method of surgery is:

A. Complete excision of membrane.
B. Partial excision of membrane, leaving a small part at the medial side.
C. Partial excision of membrane, leaving a small part at the lateral side.
D. Duodenostomy.
E. Duodenojejunostomy.

Q. 9
Regarding association of duodenal atresia, which of the following is true?

A. Down syndrome.
B. Congenital heart disease.
C. Malrotation 30 percent.
D. Annular pancreas 30 percent.
E. All the above.

Q. 10
Regarding duodenal atresia, which of the following statements is true?

A. Type III atresia is commonest.
B. Fifty per cent obstruction is below the ampulla of Vater.
C. Wind sock is variant of type I atresia.

D. Survival rate is 60 percent.
E. Almost all reported deaths are from sepsis.

Jejunal Atresia/Ileal Atresia

Q. 11
Regarding jejunal and ileal atresia, which is false?

A. Three bubble sign is a feature of jejunal atresia.
B. In ileal atresia, there are multiple air-fluid levels.
C. Jaundice is more common in ileal atresia than jejunal atresia.
D. Abdominal distension is more significant in ileal atresia than jejunal atresia.
E. Both present with abdominal distension, bilious vomiting and failure to pass meconium.

Q. 12
The apple-peel variety of jejunal atresia is:

A. Type I atresia.
B. Type II atresia.
C. Type III A atresia.
D. Type III B atresia.
E. Type IV atresia.

Meconeum Ileus

Q. 13
Complications of meconium ileus include all the following except:

A. Volvulus.
B. Perforation.

C. Peritonitis.
D. Cystic fibrosis.
E. Pseudocyst formation.

Q. 14
Regarding radiology in meconium ileus, which of the following is false?

A. Simple meconium ileus does not show air-fluid levels.
B. Calcification is seen in complicated cases.
C. There is a ground glass appearance.
D. Contrast enema shows megacolon.
E. Contrast enema shows ipsilateral pellets of meconium.

Q. 15
Which appear in the differential diagnosis of meconium ileus?

A. Total colonic aganglionosis.
B. Long-segment Hirschsprung's disease.
C. Ileal atresia.
D. Meconium plug syndrome.
E. All the above.

Q. 16
Complications of gastrografin include all the following except:

A. Constipation.
B. Perforation.
C. Pecrotising enterocolitis.
D. Shock.
E. Death.

Q. 17
Of the long-term complications of meconium ileus, which of the following is most accurate?

 A. Distal intestinal obstruction.
 B. Intussusception.
 C. Cholecystitis.
 D. Inguinal hernia.
 E. All the above.

Q. 18
Regarding cystic fibrosis, which of the following is false?

 A. Autosomal recessive.
 B. Disorder involving chromosome number 8.
 C. Defective chloride channel.
 D. Pancreatic insufficiency in about 90 percent of cases.
 E. Affects pancreatic, biliary, respiratory, gastrointestinal and reproductive systems.

Q. 19
Regarding incidence of complications of cystic fibrosis, which statement is true?

 A. Meconium ileus is more common than pancreatic insufficiency.
 B. Obstructive biliary disease is more common than meconium ileus.
 C. Azoospermia is less common than meconium ileus.
 D. Meconium ileus is more common than azoospermia.
 E. Azoospermia is more common than pancreatic insufficiency.

Q. 20
Survival of meconium ileus is:

    A. less than 90 percent.
    B. 70–80 percent.
    C. 50–60 percent.
    D. 40–50 percent.
    E. 10–20 percent.

Q. 21
Calcification with air-fluid level is feature of:

    A. Jejunal atresia.
    B. Simple meconium ileus.
    C. Complicated meconium ileus.
    D. Hirschsprung's disease.
    E. Colonic stenosis.

Q. 22
Meconium ileus is treated nonsurgically in what percentage of cases?

    A. 30 percent.
    B. 40 percent.
    C. 60 percent.
    D. 80 percent.
    E. 90 percent.

Q. 23
Regarding meconium ileus and cystic fibrosis, which is true?

    A. meconium ileus is associated with cystic fibrosis in 90 percent of cases.

B. meconium ileus occurs in 10–20 percent of patients with cystic fibrosis.
C. meconium ileus occurs in 40 percent of patients with cystic fibrosis.
D. A and B are true.
E. A and C are true.

Malrotation

Q. 24
Regarding rotation of the gut, which of the following is false?

A. Normal rotation occurs 270 degrees clockwise.
B. If rotation occurs only counterclockwise, it is called incomplete rotation.
C. Reverse rotation is 180 degrees.
D. Hyper-rotation occurs at 360 degrees or more, and caecum comes to rest in splenic flexure.
E. Rotation occurs between the eighth and twentieth weeks of gestation.

Q. 25
Regarding the management of malrotation, which one is false?

A. Plain X-rays of the abdomen show dilated colon.
B. Upper GIT contrast shows abnormal configuration of the C loop of the duodenum and the duodenojejunal junction on right side of midline.
C. Ultrasound shows inversion in a superior mesenteric artery (SMA) with superior mesenteric vein (SMV) relationship with the SMA on right side and SMV on the left.

D. Untwisting of volvulus requires about 180-degree counterclockwise rotation.

Q. 26
In Ladd's procedure, what should be avoided?

A. Restoration of intestinal anatomy in nonrotation position.
B. Division of peritoneal band.
C. Division of superior mesenteric artery.
D. Widening of mesentery.
E. Division of ligamentum trietz.

Q. 27
Gut rotational abnormalities produce all except:

A. Acute midgut volvulus.
B. Chronic midgut volvulus.
C. Acute duodenal obstruction secondary to Ladd's band.
D. Chronic duodenal obstruction secondary to congenital band.
E. Meconium ileus.

Q. 28
Normal intestinal rotation involves:

A. 270-degree counterclockwise rotation of duodenojejunal loop around the superior mesenteric artery.
B. 270-degree clockwise rotation of duodenojejunal loop around the superior mesenteric artery.
C. 270-degree counterclockwise rotation of duodenojejunal loop around the inferior mesenteric vein.

D. 360-degree counterclockwise rotation of duodenojejunal loop around the inferior mesenteric artery.
E. 180-degree counterclockwise rotation of duodenojejunal loop around superior mesenteric artery.

Q. 29
Regarding the presentation of malrotation, which is true?

A. Thirty percent presents within first week of life.
B. Fifty percent presents within first month.
C. Ninety percent presents within first year.
D. All the above are correct.
E. None of the above is correct.

Q. 30
About procedure for malrotation, which statement is true?

A. Reduction of volvulus.
B. Division of Ladd's band
C. Broadening of mesentery between duodenojejunal junction and cecum.
D. Appendectomy and placement of cecum of left side.
E. All the above.

Q. 31
Normal foetal intestinal rotation occurs:

A. Between two and four weeks gestational age.
B. Between four and ten weeks gestational age.
C. Between ten and fourteen weeks gestational age.
D. Between fourteen and sixteen weeks gestational age.
E. After sixteen weeks of gestation.

Achalasia Cardia

Q. 32
Regarding achalasia cardia, which one is false?

A. There is failure of relaxation of the lower oesophagus.
B. Histochemistry shows an increase in neuropeptide, VIP and gastrin.
C. Nifedipine and calcium channel antagonists are used as medical treatment.
D. Pneumatic dilatation is one of the treatments.
E. Myotomy over 4–5 cm is the surgical treatment.

Q. 33
Among the diagnostic tools of achalasia cardia, which of the following is true?

A. CT scan is the investigation method of choice.
B. No finding appears on plain X-rays.
C. A barium meal shows dilatation of lower oesophagus.
D. Oesophageal manometry shows pressure greater than 30 mmHg.
E. Monitoring of pH over twenty-four hours is diagnostic.

Q. 34
In surgery for achalasia cardia, which one is false?

A. Preservation of anterior vagus nerve.
B. preservation of posterior vagus nerve.
C. Incision of 4–6 cm long made in Myotomy.
D. At least 50 per cent of the circumference of oesophageal mucosa is separated from constricting muscle.
E. Avoidance of fundoplication.

Q. 35
Regarding complications of surgery for achalasia cardia, which one is false?

A. Mediastinitis is due to failure of detection of mucosal perforation.
B. Recurrence of symptoms appear if muscle is not separated at least 50 percent of circumference of oesophagus.
C. Gastroesophageal reflux (GER) occurs due to inadequate fundoplication.
D. Dysphagia for liquid develops due to tight fundoplication.
E. GER is more common than residual or recurrence of achalasia.

Intussusception

Q. 36
A six-month-old male child presents with sudden onset of excessive cry, vomiting, and bleeding per rectum. Examination shows abdominal distension and vague mass in right-lower abdomen. Stool shows redcurrant jelly appearancWhich is the most likely diagnosis?

A. Volvulus.
B. Intussusception.
C. Duplication cyst.
D. Meckel's diverticulum.
E. Mesenteric cyst.

Q. 37
Regarding intussusception management, which of the following is false?

A. In pneumatic reduction, 160–200 mm pressure is delivered.
B. Initial reduction by pneumatic or contrast is slow, but the later part is rapid.
C. The benchmark of successful reduction is reflux of contrast or air in the colon.
D. Ultrasound shows target sign on longitudinal images.
E. All the above.

Q. 38
Regarding surgical management of intussusception, which one of the following is not true?

A. Reduction is achieved by squeezing the bowel from distal to the apex.
B. Resection may be necessary if intussusception is not reduced.
C. Resection is not necessary if the bowel is necrotic.
D. Resection may be necessary if lead point, such as Meckel's diverticulum or duplication.
E. Resection may be necessary if there is small bowel perforation.

Q. 39
Recurrence rate after pneumatic reduction is:

A. 3 percent.
B. 10 percent.
C. 20 percent.

D. 40 percent.
E. 50 percent.

Q. 40
Regarding aetiology of intussusception which one is false?

A. Aetiology is unclear in most cases.
B. Appendix may be the lead point.
C. Cystic fibrosis is present.
D. All of the above are true.
E. None of the above is true.

Vitellointestinal Duct Anomalies

Q. 41
Regarding presentation of vitellointestinal duct anomalies, the following are false except:

A. Presents as intestinal obstruction when ectopic gastric mucosa.
B. Presents with melena when there is Meckel's diverticulum with band.
C. presents with abdominal pain, mass and redcurrant jelly in stool when patent intestinal duct.
D. Presents with shiny, spherical and deep nodule in the depth of umbilical cicatrix, when prolapse of patent vitellointestinal tract.
E. Presents with features of appendicitis, when there is diverticulitis.

Q. 42
What type of discharge at umbilicus in patent/persistent vitellointestinal duct?

    A. Air and faeces.
    B. Pus.
    C. Blood.
    D. Urine.
    E. Gastric contents.

Q. 43
Regarding skin incision in different vitellointestinal duct anomalies, which of the following is the best answer?

    A. Supra-umbilical transverse incision.
    B. Infra-umbilical transverse incision.
    C. Incision at the level of umbilicus.
    D. All of the above.
    E. Non of the above.

Q. 44
Regarding urachus, all are true except:

    A. Connects midgut to yolk sac.
    B. Normally obliterates.
    C. Remnant forms median umbilical ligaments.
    D. Pathological conditions includes patent urachus, sinus and cyst.
    E. If not obliterated, leads to urine discharge from umbilicus.

Q. 45
Remnant of structures related to development of umbilicus, which of the following is false?

A. Falciform is the remnant of the umbilical vein.
B. Lateral umbilical ligament is the remnant of the omphalomesenteric vein.
C. Meckel's diverticulum is the remnant of the omphalomesenteric duct.
D. Median umbilical ligament is the remnant of the urachus.
E. Fibrous band to the umbilicus is the remnant of the omphalomesenteric arteries.

Q. 46
Uses of umbilicus include all except:

A. Cannula for umbilical vein.
B. Site for laparoscopic equipment.
C. Incision site for pyloromyotomy.
D. Exit site for stoma and urinary diversion.
E. All of the above.

Q. 47
Regarding Meckel's diverticulum, which of the following is true?

A. It is an uncommon congenital anomaly of GIT.
B. It is caused by regression of vitelline duct.
C. Blood supply is from paired vitelline arteries that originate from the aorta.

D. Pancreatic mucosa is more commonly found than gastric mucosa.
E. May develop Richter's hernia.

Q. 48
Regarding Meckel's diverticulum, which of the following is false?

A. Two per cent incidence.
B. Two types of heterogeneous mucosa.
C. Located within two inches of ileocecal valve.
D. About two inches in length.
E. Usually symptomatic within two years of age.

Q. 49
Regarding the use of Technetium scan in detecting Meckel's diverticulum, which of the following is false?

A. It is useful in detecting heterogeneous gastric mucosa.
B. Sensitivity is less than specificity.
C. Glucagon decreases the efficacy of scanning.
D. Nasogastric suction and catheterization may increase the yield of scanning.
E. False positive results may be due to duplication cyst.

Q. 50
Regarding management of Meckel's diverticulum, which of the following is false?

A. After excision of diverticulum, having two layer closure of ileum is preferable.
B. The feeding artery should be ligated.

C. If carcinoid has developed, there is greater potential for metastasis than for appendicular carcinoma.
D. In case of carcinoid development, aggressive surgical management of tumours larger than 5 cm is recommended.
E. If left intact, the lifetime risk of complication is 2 percent.

Omphalocele and Gastroschisis

Q. 51
In omphalocele major, which of the following is less toxic, if used to induce eschar formation?

A. Alcohol.
B. Iodine
C. Mercury-containing compound.
D. Mercurochrome.
E. Silver sulfadiazine.

Q. 52
For omphalocele minor, which one is the best option?

A. Primary repair.
B. Development of ventral hernia.
C. Staged repair.
D. Silo application.
E. Utilisation of prosthesis for closure of facial defect over polyethylene or silastic sheath.

Q. 53
Omphalocele differ from gastroschisis in all except:

A. Herniated contents may include stomach and liver.
B. Occurs at right to umbilicus.
C. Umbilicus is attached at the tip.
D. More likely associated with a congenital defect, such as cardiac defect or Down syndrome
E. Less likely associated with gut atresia.

Q. 54
Ideal treatment for omphalocele is:

A. Primary closure.
B. SILO placement.
C. DECRO (delayed external compression and reduction).
D. Mobilisation of large skin flap and skin closure only.
E. Placement of prosthetic material and closure of skin over this material, with serial reduction of this prosthetic material.

Q. 55
Omphalocele differs from gastroschisis in all except:

A. Location.
B. Size of defect.
C. Presence of sac.
D. Cord attachment.
E. Malrotation.

Q. 56
Regarding omphalocele, all are true except:

A. Develops because of involution of right umbilical vein, which may leave a week area.
B. Develops because of failure of closure of body wall by cephalic, caudal and lateral folds.
C. Develops because of poor development of abdominal cavity that leads failure of reduction of physiological hernia.
D. Associated with pentalogy of Cantrell.
E. Associated with trisomy syndrome.

Q. 57
Immediate management of gastroschisis includes all except:

A. Nasogastric tube.
B. Folly's catheterization.
C. Places on side/lateral position.
D. Intravenous fluid.
E. Vitamin D.

Q. 58
The following agents can be used as sclerosing agent for topical application for non-operative treatment of Exomphalos, except.

A. Mercurochrome.
B. Silver sulphadiazine.
C. Ten per cent silver nitrate solution.
D. Seventy per cent alcohol.
E. Biological dressing.

Q. 59
The following are the late complications of gastroschisis repair except:

A. Growth delay.
B. Low IQ.
C. Necrotising enterocolitis.
D. Atypical appendicitis.
E. Intestinal obstruction.

Q. 60
Studies related to gastroschisis shows the following except:

A. Incidence is 1.5–2.5 percent per 10,000.
B. Complete primary closure can be performed in 20 percent of cases.
C. Mortality rate is about 5–10 percent of cases.
D. Associated intestinal atresia is 5–25 percent of cases.
E. Some need fundoplication following abdominal wall repair.

Q. 61
Regarding gastroschisis, which of the following statements is true?

A. Intestinal atresia is seen in 10 percent of cases.
B. The mean time from operation to initiation of oral feed is 3–6 weeks.
C. The most common late complication is adhesive small bowel obstruction.
D. All of the above are true.
E. All of the above are false.

Q. 62
Gastroschisis is associated with malrotation, but volvulus is a very rare event because:

A. No band.
B. Short mesentery.
C. Wide mesentery.
D. Adhesion formation.
E. Fixation during gastroschisis repair.

Q. 63
The most common cardiovascular malformation associated with exomphalos is:

A. Atrial septal defect.
B. Ventricular septal defect.
C. Transposition of great vessels.
D. Tetralogy of Fallot.
E. None of the above.

Q. 64
The position of defect in relation to umbilicus in gastroschisis is:

A. The defect is to the right of the umbilicus.
B. The defect is to the left of the umbilicus.
C. The defect is under the umbilicus.
D. The defect is above the umbilicus.
E. The defect is in the umbilicus.

Ascites

Q. 65
Causes of biliary ascites include all except:

A. Congenital hepatic fibrosis.
B. Traumatic perforation of the bile duct.
C. Spontaneous perforation of common bile duct secondary to distal duct obstruction.
D. Spontaneous perforation of common bile duct secondary to pancreatic juice reflux up to the common bile duct.
E. Biliary atresia.

Q. 66
Causes of hepatocellular ascites include all except:

A. Glycogen storage disease.
B. Lysosomal storage disease.
C. Galactosemia.
D. Antitrypsin deficiency.
E. Atresia or stenosis of major lacteal at base of mesentery or cisterna chyli.

Q. 67
Features of urinary ascites on laboratory analysis of ascites include all except:

A. Creatinine 5–10 mg per 100 ml.
B. PH <7.0.
C. Albumin 2–3 G per 100 ml.
D. Triglyceride <50 mg per 100 ml.
E. Bilirubin <1 mg per 100 ml.

Q. 68
The following are treatment options of urinary ascites except:

A. Peritoneal drain.
B. Folly's catheter.
C. Valve ablation in posterior urethral valve.
D. Peritoneovenous shunt.
E. Percutaneous nephrostomy.

Trichobezoar

Q. 69
Collection of which of the following in stomach is called trichobezoar?

A. Seeds.
B. Needles.
C. Threads.
D. Medications.
E. Hairs.

SECTION 2

ABDOMEN B

Pancreas

Q. 1
Regarding the development of the pancreas, which is true?

    A. Ventral bud forms most of pancreas.
    B. If dorsal bud does not rotate forward, the condition is called annular pancreas.
    C. Normally duct of Santorini becomes major duct in the end.
    D. In pancreatic divisum, duct of wirsung is the major duct.
    E. Dorsal bud forms head, body and tail of pancreas.

Q. 2
Regarding the anatomy of the pancreas, which is true?

    A. Head at the level of L3, body at the level of L2 and tail at the level of L1.

B. Anatomical continuity is established by peritoneal reflection.
C. Venous drainage to inferior mesenteric vein.
D. All above.
E. None above.

Q. 3
Regarding cause of pancreatitis, which one is most appropriate answer?

A. Mumps.
B. ERCP.
C. Choledochal cyst.
D. All of the above.
E. None of the above.

Q. 4
For the diagnosis of acute pancreatitis, which is false?

A. Serum amylase is specific to pancreatitis.
B. Serum amylase peaks within 48 hours.
C. Plain radiograph shows epigastric haziness and colonic cut-off sign.
D. CT scan can detect pancreatic anomalies.
E. ERCP is rarely indicated.

Q. 5
Regarding the treatment of pancreatitis, which is true?

A. Morphine is better than Meperidine.
B. Total parenteral nutrition is not helpful.
C. Glucagon is not helpful.

D. Surgical intervention is required if diagnosis is uncertain.
E. Repeated surgical drainage is not controversial.

Q. 6
In chronic relapsing pancreatitis, which is false?

A. Recurrent lower abdominal pain occurs.
B. Crohn's disease is one of the causes.
C. Pancreatic calcification is diagnostic for chronic pancreatitis.
D. ERCP may shows stenotic papilla of Vater.
E. Pancreaticojejunostomy is one of the surgical option.

Q. 7
Regarding pseudo-pancreatic cyst, which is false?

A. It develops after pancreatic injury.
B. The cyst lies mostly in lesser sac.
C. The cyst lined by epithelium.
D. Cystic fluid is clear or straw colour.
E. Serum amylase is as high as 50,000/ml.

Q. 8
Regarding management of pseudo-pancreatic cyst, which is false?

A. Abdominal pain is the most common symptom.
B. Mass may be palpable in epigastrium.
C. Ultrasound and CT gives accurate diagnosis.
D. Medical management and supportive treatment for three weeks.
E. Recurrence in children is low as compared to adults.

Q. 9
In infantile hyperinsulism, all are true except:

A. Insulin level is >10 micro unites/ml.
B. Glucose level is <50 mg/dl.
C. Diazoxide helps by acting as beta-cells specific cytotoxic agents.
D. Surgical treatment to prevent hypoglycaemia brain damage.
E. Operation requires 95 per cent resection of pancreas.

Q. 10
Regarding Ranson criteria for pancreatitis during first 48 hours, all of the following are true except:

A. White cells more than 16,000.
B. Ten per cent decrease in haematocrit.
C. Increase in blood urea nitrogen more than 5.
D. Serum calcium less than 8 mg/dl
E. Fluid sequestration more than 6 L.

Portal Hypertension

Q. 11
In management of portal hypertension, which of the following is false?

A. In endoscopic variceal ligation, the band and varices slough off in 5–7 days.
B. In proximal splenorenal shunt, splenectomy is required.
C. In portocaval shunt, side of portal vein and end of inferior vena cava is anastomosed.

D. In children, mesocaval and splenorenal shunts are commonly performed.
E. In mesocaval shunt inferior mesenteric vein is dissected 5 cm inferior to the pancreas.

Biliary Atresia

Q. 12
Regarding type and classification of biliary atresia, which of the following is false?

A. Type I atresia at porta is the most common.
B. Type I is the obliteration of the common bile duct, while the proximal bile ducts are patent.
C. Type IIa is atresia of the hepatic duct, with cystic bile ducts found at the porta hepatis.
D. Type IIb is atresia of the cystic duct, common bile duct, and hepatic ducts.
E. Type III is involvement of the extrahepatic biliary tree and intrahepatic ducts of the porta hepatis.

Q. 13
Regarding cause of biliary atresia, which is true?

A. True cause is still unknown.
B. Failure of extrahepatic and intrahepatic duct system to meet.
C. Environmental factors.
D. Viral infection.
E. All of the above.

Q. 14
Regarding presentation of biliary atresia, which is true?

A. Most infants are preterm.
B. Classical triad is abdominal pain, abdominal mass, and jaundice.
C. The earlier the presentation, the better the prognosis.
D. The child never presents with hepatic decompensation.
E. Clear urine and dark stool are commonly seen.

Q. 15
In preoperative management of biliary atresia, what is not required?

A. Choleretics.
B. Antibiotic.
C. Upper GIT contrast study.
D. Metabolic and nutritional care.
E. Essential fatty acid supplement.

Q. 16
All are true regarding surgical technique in biliary atresia except:

A. Roux-en-Y with intussuscepted valve reduces the chances of cholangitis.
B. Modification by shortening the loop of Roux-en-Y reduces the chances of cholangitis.
C. Roux-en-Y is the operation for non-correctable type.
D. Roux-en-Y is the operation for correctable type.
E. Modification by Kasai's procedure is for prevention of cholangitis.

Q. 17
Select the best answer about the causes/cause of cholangitis after surgery for biliary atresia.

    A. Portal venous infection.
    B. destruction of lymphatics at porta hepatitis.
    C. bacterial translocation.
    D. all of the above.
    E. none of the above.

Q. 18
Regarding complications of surgery for biliary atresia, which of the following statements is false?

    A. Cholangitis.
    B. Portal hypotension.
    C. Stricture of anastomosis.
    D. Leakage of anastomosis and peritonitis.
    E. Non of the above.

Q. 19
The best answer among following regarding differential diagnosis of biliary atresia is:

    A. Biliary hypoplasia.
    B. Choledochal cyst.
    C. Inspissated bile syndrome.
    D. Neonatal jaundice.
    E. All of the above.

Q. 20
Regarding management of biliary atresia, which of the following is false?

A. Pre-operative presence of gallbladder is an indication of cholangiography.
B. Preoperative gallbladder is used as guide.
C. In Roux-en-Y portoenterostomy, a 20 cm Roux-en-Y loop, 10 cm distal to duodenojejunal junction is used.
D. Pre-operative biopsy is taken from right lobe.
E. If biopsy shows ductules >150 micro-m, this indicates a good prognosis.

Q. 21
Regarding complication and survival of biliary atresia, which of the following is false?

A. Hepatic fibrosis stops once achievement of good biliary drainage.
B. Early cholangitis after portoenterostomy is noted in more than 20 percent of cases.
C. Portal hypertension is seen in more than 50 percent of cases.
D. Survival after liver transplantation is better than surgery for biliary atresia.
E. There is relationship between the age at which portoenterostomy is performed and restoration of bile flow.

Q. 22
After portoenterostomy for biliary atresia, which one of the following statements is false?

    A. Most patients require liver transplantation within three years.
    B. The patients who survive following Kasai portoenterostomy remain free of jaundice for 5–10 years.
    C. Portoenterostomy provides long-term biliary drainage in about one-third of patients.
    D. Cholangitis is the most common complication.
    E. Age of the patient is the most common predictor of long-term outcome.

Q. 23
Ultrasound finding of biliary atresia is:

    A. Doughnut sign.
    B. Triangular cord sign.
    C. Sandwich sign.
    D. None of the above.
    E. All of the above.

Choledochal Cyst

Q. 24
Regarding classification of choledochal cyst, which of the following is false?

    A. Fusiform dilatation of extrahepatic duct is the commonest variety.
    B. Type II is the diverticulum of extrahepatic duct.

C. Type III cysts are choledochocele, dilations of the distal common bile duct located either in the duodenal wall, or the head of the pancreas.
D. Type IV choledochal cysts are similar in appearance to the extrahepatic ducts of the type I choledochal cysts with the addition of intrahepatic biliary duct dilation.
E. Caroli's disease is the other name for the type I variety of cyst.

Q. 25
Regarding aetiology of choledochocele, which is true?

A. Reflux of pancreatic enzyme in proximal biliary duct.
B. Obstruction of distal duct.
C. Congenital weakness of wall of duct.
D. All of the above are true.
E. All of the above are false.

Q. 26
Regarding diagnosis of choledochal cyst, which of the following is true?

A. Adult form occurs in children older than 7 years.
B. Classical trait is acholic stool, jaundice and hepatomegaly.
C. Infantile form occurs in 1 to 3 months of age.
D. High serum unconjugated bilirubin.
E. Per-operative liver biopsy is not indicated.

Q. 27
The most common surgical procedure for choledochal cyst is:

A. Cystoduodenostomy.
B. Roux-en-Y cystojejunostomy.

C. Cyst excision with Roux-en-Y hepaticojejunostomy.
D. End-to-side Roux-en-Y choledochojejunostomy.
E. Longitudinal duodenoscopy for choledochocele.

Q. 28

Regarding post-operative complication of choledochal cyst, which is false?

A. Pancreatitis is seen more common after type I choledochal cyst surgery.
B. Cholangiocarcinoma is known complication.
C. Severe GIT bleeding occurs.
D. Pancreatic duct or bile duct stone occurs.
E. Incidence of cholangitis is reduced by making long jejunal loop and use of choleretics.

Q. 29

With regard to choledochal cyst, which of the following is not true?

A. Radio-isotope studies show a delayed excretion of radioisotope from the liver, a dilated common bile duct and retarded drainage into the bowel.
B. Jaundice is always at the time of presentation.
C. Patients have variable presentation.
D. Patient may be asymptomatic.
E. Squamous cell carcinoma is the most common histological variant that can occur.

Splenectomy

Q. 30
Regarding splenectomy, all of the following are false except:

A. Electrocoagulation should not be used to achieve haemostasis.
B. Subcostal incision is preferred over midline incision for splenectomy after trauma.
C. Squeeze spleen gently to return as much blood as possible before clamping vessels.
D. Splenic vein should be clamped before artery.
E. Posterior peritoneum and fascia is closed by non-absorbable suture.

Q. 31
For overwhelming post-splenectomy infection, which of the following is false?

A. Mortality rate is 25 percent.
B. It is caused by pneumococcus (most common), Haemophilus influenzae, and meningococcus.
C. Risk is high in children less than 5 years of age.
D. It is more common in first two years after splenectomy.
E. It is more common in children undergoes elective splenectomy for haematological disease.

Hirschsprung's Disease

Q. 32
Regarding aetiology of Hirschsprung's disease, all are true except:

    A. Failure of migration of neural crest cells.
    B. Absence of neural crest cell adhesion molecule.
    C. Decrease expression of class II antigen in mucosa and submucosa.
    D. Mutation and deletion at chromosome number 10.
    E. Deficiency nitrous oxide synthetase.

Q. 33
Regarding nervous system of intestine in Hirschsprung's disease, all are false except:

    A. Adrenergic, which is normally inhibitory, also becomes excitatory.
    B. Excess of ganglion cells.
    C. Atrophy of nerve bundle.
    D. Increased extrinsic innervation.
    E. Inhibitory cholinergic.

Q. 34
A barium enema shows the following findings on Hirschsprung's disease except:

    A. Spastic (narrow) distal intestine with dilated proximal intestine.
    B. Transitional zone.
    C. Presacral space.
    D. Right-sided sigmoid colon
    E. Increased recto-sigmoid index.

Q. 35
Differential diagnosis of Hirschsprung's disease include all except:

   A. Meconium ileus.
   B. Distal ileal or colonic atresia.
   C. Small left colon syndrome.
   D. Hyperthyroidism.
   E. Intestinal Neuronal dysplasia.

Q. 36
What is not true about the surgical procedures of Hirschsprung's disease?

   A. In Duhamel procedure, there is retro-rectal pull-through.
   B. In Swenson procedure, there is resection and anastomosis.
   C. In Soave procedure, there is endo-rectal pull-through.
   D. Martin's modification is for ultra-short segment Hirschsprung's disease.
   E. Aganglionic patch is used in Kimura's procedure.

Q. 37
What is false about complications of surgical procedures of Hirschsprung's disease?

   A. Faecal soiling.
   B. Incontinence.
   C. Residual Hirschsprung's disease.
   D. All of the above.
   E. None of the above.

Q. 38
Which is true about full thickness rectal biopsy for Hirschsprung's disease?

A. It is an established manner of diagnosis.
B. It is taken from below the dentate line.
C. It is taken from anterior rectal wall.
D. Rectal defect is left open.
E. Stay suture helps in taken biopsy, should be avoided.

Q. 39
Which of the following is false for levelling colostomy for Hirschsprung's disease?

A. You should determine the ganglionic level at the time of colostomy.
B. It facilitates subsequent pull–through.
C. It allows proximal bowel to grow, which will stretch the mesentery and simply subsequent pull-through procedure.
D. All above.
E. None of the above.

Q. 40
Which of the following is not true regarding colostomy for Hirschsprung's disease?

A. It is easy to identify the transitional zone in neonate.
B. On the frozen section, hypertrophy of nerve bundle, despite of presence of ganglion, suggests that one is still in the transitional zone.
C. Loop colostomy is created at one of the normal biopsy site.

D. Aganglionosis of appendix indicates total colonic aganglionosis.
E. Stoma usually starts to act within 24 hours.

Q. 41
Regarding rectal suction biopsy, for Hirschsprung's disease, which of the following is false?

A. It is a painless procedure, provided it is taken at least 2.5 cm above the anal verge in neonates and 3.5 cm in older children.
B. Pressure usually used is above 300 mm Hg.
C. Specimen is usually taken from anterior wall.
D. Specimen is usually 3 mm long and 1 mm wide.
E. Inadequate specimen is a common problem.

Q. 42
Causes of constipation in children include all except:

A. Anteriorly placed anus.
B. Anal stenosis.
C. Anal fissure.
D. Cystic fibrosis.
E. Hyperthyroidism.

Q. 43
Regarding Hirschsprung's disease and its features, which of the following statements is not true?

A. It is mostly seen in boys.
B. Most patients are diagnosed before one year of age.
C. Most patients are preterm.
D. Abdominal distension is a common finding.

E. Level of disease is mostly recto-sigmoid.

Q. 44
Risk of Hirschsprung's disease in future children is:

A. Less than 10 percent.
B. 20–30 percent.
C. 30–40 percent.
D. 40–50 percent.
E. More than 50 percent.

Q. 45
Incidence of stricture formation after pull-through procedure in Hirschsprung's disease is:

A. 1 to 4 percent.
B. 4–8 percent.
C. 8–12 percent.
D. 12–16 percent.
E. more than 16 percent.

Q. 46
The most common late complication in Hirschsprung's disease is:

A. Constipation.
B. Diarrhoea.
C. Enterocolitis.
D. Stricture.
E. Perforation.

Q. 47
What percentage of Hirschsprung's disease associated with Down syndrome?

A. 1–2 percent.
B. 2–3 percent.
C. 4–5 percent.
D. 5–6 percent.
E. 7–8 percent.

Q. 48
Regarding types of Hirschsprung's disease according to involved segments, which of the following statements is false?

A. In short segment disease, rectal and distal sigmoid colonic involvement only occurs.
B. Long segment typically extends to splenic flexure/ transverse colon.
C. In total colonic aganglionosis, occasional there is extension of aganglionosis into small bowel.
D. Ultrashort segment disease is 3–4 cm of internal anal sphincter only.
E. All of the above are false.

Q. 49
What percentage of Hirschsprung's disease is associated with meconium plug syndrome?

A. 10–30 percent.
B. 30–40 percent.
C. 40–50 percent.
D. 50–60 percent.
E. None of the above.

Anorectal Malformation

Q. 50
Among different anorectal malformation, which of the following condition does not needs colostomy?

    A. Perineal fistula.
    B. Rectourethral fistula.
    C. Rectovesical fistula.
    D. Imperforated anus without fistula.
    E. Rectal atresia.

Q. 51
In the girls with anorectal malformation, which of the following conditions is the most common?

    A. Rectovesical fistula.
    B. Rectovestibular fistula.
    C. Rectovaginal fistula.
    D. Rectourethral fistula.
    E. Common cloaca.

Q. 52
Which of the following is not a feature of low imperforate anus?

    A. Skin tag.
    B. Bucket-handle malformation.
    C. Anal dimple.
    D. Flat perineum.
    E. Perineal fistula.

Q. 53
What is false about the levatorani muscle?

A. Normally the rectum is surrounded laterally and posteriorly by levatorani muscle mechanism.
B. In imperforate anus with recto-vesical fistula, levatorani lies posterior and lateral to rectum.
C. When levator ani contracts, it pushes the rectum forward.
D. All of the above are true.
E. All of the above are false.

Q. 54
In persistent cloaca, a common channel of what length has poor sphincter mechanism?

A. >0.5 cm.
B. >1 cm.
C. >1 cm
D. >2 cm.
E. >3 cm.

Q. 55
In male neonates with anorectal malformation, clinical evidence is present on perineal inspection in what percentage of cases?

A. 50 percent.
B. 60 percent.
C. 70 percent.
D. 80 percent.
E. 90 percent.

Q. 56
In boys, the definitive procedure of intermediate type of imperforate anus is:

A. Anoplasty
B. Colostomy.
C. Posterior sagittal anoplasty.
D. Posterior sagittal anorectoplasty (PSARP).
E. Anal repositioning.

Q. 57
Disadvantage of transverse colostomy, in comparison to descending colostomy in imperforate anus include all except:

A. Long segment is available for mobilization at the time of definitive procedure.
B. Metabolic acidosis and constipation.
C. Increased fluid and electrolyte loss.
D. Distal part difficult to wash.
E. Increased incidence of UTI, if fistula.

Q. 58
The goal of surgery in persistent cloaca include all except:

A. Separation of rectum from vagina.
B. Separation of vagina from urethra.
C. Placement of rectum within sphincter mechanism.
D. Opening of vagina in its normal location.
E. Reconstruction of old common channel as a neo-vagina.

Q. 59
In a post-operative child with anorectal malformation, which of the following is true?

A. Dilatation is started on the second month.
B. A baby pushing during each bowel movement indicates that there is some feeling during defecation process, has good prognosis.
C. Few patients have functional disorder.
D. Gas during defecation is not felt by most of patients.
E. Loss of recto-sigmoid has good prognosis.

Q. 60
High type anorectal malformation includes all except:

A. Anorectal agenesis with recto-urethral fistula.
B. Anorectal agenesis with rectovaginal fistula.
C. Anorectal agenesis without fistula.
D. Anocutaneous fistula.
E. Aectal atresia.

Q. 61
Features of high anomaly in anorectal malformation include all except:

A. Flat premium.
B. Little musculature.
C. Long sacrum.
D. Recto-vestibular fistula.
E. Rectovaginal fistula.

Q. 62
For the child with high-type imperforate anus with colostomy, the most important investigation required before definitive procedure is:

A. MRI.
B. CT scan.
C. Distal colostogram.
D. Micturating cystourethrogram (MCUG).
E. Renal ultrasound.

Necrotising Enterocolitis

Q. 63
Which of the following are management options for necrotizing enterocolitis?

A. Conservative management.
B. Peritoneal drain
C. Resection and primary anastomosis.
D. Resection with proximal ostomy and distal fistula.
E. All of the above.

Q. 64
Regarding complications of necrotizing enterocolitis, which of the following is false?

A. Terminal ileum is the most common site for stricture formation.
B. Short bowel syndrome if significant bowel is resected.
C. Cholestatic liver disease.

D. Neurodevelopment is affected in 50 percent of children who survive.
E. There is a chance of recurrent necrotizing enterocolitis.

Q. 65
The following are preventive measures for necrotizing enterocolitis except:

A. Bottle feed.
B. Infection control.
C. Immunoglobulin supplement.
D. Maternal corticosteroid therapy.
E. Use of inflammatory mediator antagonist.

Q. 66
Causes of necrotizing enterocolitis (NEC) include all except:

A. Prematurity.
B. Broad-spectrum antibiotics.
C. Formula feed.
D. Poor peristalsis.
E. Immunoglobulin administration.

Q. 67
Laboratory findings in necrotizing enterocolitis (NEC) include all except:

A. Metabolic alkalosis.
B. Neutropenia.
C. Thrombocytopenia.
D. Breath hydrogen excretion test.
E. Positive blood culture.

Q. 68
X-ray findings in NEC include all except:

A. Ileus pattern.
B. Pneumatosis intestinalis.
C. Mesenteric vein gas.
D. Pneumoperitoneum.
E. Persistent dilated loop.

Q. 69
Possible indications for operation in NEC include all except:

A. Clinical deterioration despite aggressive supportive treatment.
B. Erythema of abdominal wall.
C. Abdominal mass.
D. Positive blood culture.
E. Portal vein gas.

Antegrade Continent Catheterizable Stoma

Q. 70
Of Melon's procedure (catheterizable stoma for chronic faecal problem), which of the following is false?

A. It is retrograde continent catheterizable colonic stoma.
B. Stoma is used for colonic washout.
C. For wheelchair-bound patients, higher site of stoma is more suitable.
D. For mobile patients, stoma is best sited in the right iliac fossa.
E. It is used in neuropathy with chronic constipation.

Q. 71
In continent catheterizable stoma, which of the following is false?

A. Appendix is mobilized on its vascular pedicle.
B. Caecal submucosal tunnel about 5 cm.
C. Appendix may be re-implanted in either in peristaltic and antiperistaltic fashion.
D. Bowel preparation is required before operation.
E. Success rate is about 50 per cent.

Q. 72
Using appendix in Melon's procedure (antegrade continent catheterizable stoma), which is the least likely complication?

A. Stenosis.
B. Retraction.
C. Leakage.
D. Prolapse.
E. Enema fails to pass through rectum.

Q. 73
Which of the following is false for ante-grade continent catheterizable stoma for faecal incontinence?

A. Bowel preparation is required.
B. In wheelchair-bound patients, a low site of stoma is usually required.
C. When using appendix, after amputation, a caecal submucosal tunnel of about 5 cm is created.
D. Appendix may be re-implanted in peristaltic and antiperistalsis fashion.
E. After administration of fluid for ante-grade enema, evacuation usually starts in 15 minutes.

Rectal Prolapse

Q. 74
Best answer among following for precipitating factor causing rectal prolapse is:

   A. Diarrhoea.
   B. Constipation.
   C. Too early or overzealous toilet training.
   D. All of the above.
   E. None of the above.

Q. 75
Non-operative management of rectal prolapse includes:

   A. Correction of bowel habit.
   B. Diet containing more vegetable and cereal fibres.
   C. Ensuring defecation is prompt and quick and performed in sitting position.
   D. Temporary support by finger and prolonged support by stripping of buttock together.
   E. All of the above.

Q. 76
Regarding operative treatment of rectal prolapse, which of the following is true?

   A. Submucosal sclerotherapy is given in lateral and anterior direction.
   B. In the Thiersch procedure, three incisions (3, 7 and 11 o'clock positions) are required.
   C. Recurrence rate is 10–20 percent.

D. Injection sclerotherapy should not be repeated.
E. Internal fixation by laparotomy is an option.

Q. 77
What number of patients with cystic fibrosis have rectal prolapse?

A. All.
B. Half.
C. One-third.
D. One-fifth.
E. One-eighth.

Ulcerative Colitis

Q. 78
Regarding ulcerative colitis, all of the following are false except:

A. It is not an immunological response to bacterial or chemical agent.
B. It is an inflammatory condition of rectal and colonic muscle.
C. The rectum is involved in 50 percent of cases.
D. Inflammation extends proximally in a contiguous manner.
E. Macroscopically, it has a cobblestone appearance.

Q. 79
Regarding extraintestinal manifestation of ulcerative colitis, which of the following is false?

A. Conjunctivitis.
B. Pyoderma Gangrenosum.
C. Erythema Nodosum.
D. Sclerosing cholangitis.
E. Arthralgia.

Q. 80
Colonic features on barium enema in ulcerative colitis include all except:

A. Colon is shortened.
B. Colon is narrow.
C. Colon is rigid.
D. Extensive haustral fold.
E. Extensive formation of pseudo polyp.

Q. 81
Regarding treatment of ulcerative colitis, which of the following is false?

A. Corticosteroid for 2–3 months; may induce remission.
B. Persistent symptoms despite of medical therapy is an indication of surgery.
C. Growth retardation is an indication of surgery.
D. Surgical treatment option is distal colostomy.
E. Cleaning enema is avoided before surgery.

Q. 82
Regarding ulcerative colitis, which of the following statements is false?

A. Joint is involved in 20–25 percent of cases.
B. Principal treatment is steroid and amino salicylate.
C. Indication of colostomy is intractable disease.
D. Azathioprine response time is 7 days.
E. Operative mortality is about 1 percent.

Crohn's Disease

Q. 83
Regarding Crohn's disease, which of the following is true?

A. Microscopically, it has a cobblestone appearance.
B. Granuloma has caseation.
C. Inflammation limited to mucosa.
D. Skip lesions are common.
E. In 20 percent of cases, both small and large bowel are involved.

Q. 84
The following are features of Crohn's disease except:

A. Vague abdominal pain.
B. String sign of Kantor in upper GIT series.
C. Joint swelling as extraintestinal manifestation.
D. Disease progress leading to stricture formation.
E. Endoscopy showing pseudo polyp.

Q. 85
In Crohn's disease, surgical treatment is indicated in all of the following except:

  A. Intestinal obstruction.
  B. Toxic megacolon.
  C. Massive haemorrhage.
  D. Perforation.
  E. Fistula.

Q. 86
Which one is the most common complication of Crohn's disease?

  A. Intestinal stenosis.
  B. Septicaemia.
  C. Severe bleeding.
  D. Fistula formation.
  E. Free perforation of colon.

Q. 87
Regarding the prognosis of Crohn's disease, which one is false?

  A. Recurrence after resection is uncommon.
  B. Recurrence after surgery may lead to further surgery.
  C. Improvement in lifestyle is critical.
  D. Most achieve normal height and weight.
  E. Mortality is low.

Q. 88
With regard to Crohn's disease, all of the below are true except:

A. Perianal fistula and abscess are the first signs of disease.
B. Perianal disease occurs later than intestinal manifestations.
C. Oral metronidazole gives good response in a number of cases.
D. The mainstay of initial medical therapy is treatment with corticosteroid.
E. Stoma should be avoided in Crohn's disease.

SECTION 3

ABDOMEN C

Inguinal Hernia

Q. 1
Contralateral exploration is indicated in inguinal hernia in all of the following conditions, except:

    A. Anterior abdominal wall disorder.
    B. Girls under two years of age with right-sided hernia.
    C. When second anaesthesia is considered at high risk.
    D. Down syndrome.
    E. When it would be difficult for patient to travel.

Q. 2
Which of the following is called Litter's hernia?

    A. Obstructed.
    B. When blood supply is compromised.
    C. When double loop in the sac.
    D. When Meckel's diverticulum is the content of sac.

E. When portion of circumference of small bowel is strangulated.

Q. 3
Causes of recurrence of hernia include all except:

A. Operation on incarcerated hernia.
B. Tearing of friable sac.
C. Failure of complete ligation of sac.
D. Ligation of sac at internal ring.
E. Concomitant disease.

Q. 4
In a female child, what percentage of cases hernial sac contains salpinx?

A. Less than 5 percent.
B. 5–10 percent.
C. 10–15 percent.
D. 15–20 percent.
E. 20–25 percent.

Q. 5
Regarding inguinal hernia, which of the following statements is false?

A. Testicular atrophy has been reported in 3–5 percent of boys following incarceration.
B. Twin boys has 10 per cent incidence of inguinal hernia.
C. Child with ventriculoperitoneal shunt has 15 percent incidence of inguinal hernia.
D. Premature infant with post conceptual age of 55 weeks does not requires in hospital monitoring.

E. Transillumination differentiates inguinal hernia from hydrocele.

Umbilical Hernia

Q. 6
What is false about umbilical hernia?

A. It is common in girls.
B. It is usually operated by a curved incision below the umbilicus.
C. Surgery is indicated if not closed after 2 years.
D. When the defect is more than 2 cm, it is also an indication of surgery.
E. All of the above are false.

Q. 7
What percentage of umbilical hernia closes spontaneously?

A. 20 percent.
B. 30 percent.
C. 40 percent.
D. 60 percent.
E. 80 percent.

Q. 8
Regarding umbilical hernia, which of the following statements is false?

A. It occurs about 26 percent of African American children.
B. Size of defect has direct relationship to spontaneous closure.

C. Umbilical hernia is classified as hernia with small defect if defect is less than 3 cm.
D. The frequency of repair is more common in large hernia.
E. Incarceration and strangulation is not common.

Circumcision

Q. 9
Which of the following is the commonest reason of circumcision in the world?

A. Religious reasons.
B. Social reasons.
C. Urinary tract infection.
D. Phimosis.
E. Para-phimosis.

Q. 10
The following are complications of circumcisions except:

A. Haemorrhage.
B. Dilated meatus.
C. Sepsis.
D. Fistula formation.
E. Excision of too much or too little skin.

Bleeding Per Rectum

Q. 11
Intussusception is common among which age group?

A. Neonates.
B. Infants.

C. Toddlers.
D. Preschool.
E. Teenagers.

Q. 12
Regarding Peutz–Jeghers syndrome, which is false?

A. Polyps from the stomach to rectum.
B. Most of the polyps are in the small intestine.
C. Autosomal dominant.
D. If not treated becomes malignant in 20 per cent of cases.
E. Sometimes has isolated juvenile polyp.

Q. 13
Regarding familial adenomatous polyposis, which of the following is false?

A. Autosomal recessive.
B. Mutation at long arm of chromosome number 5.
C. Nearly all untreated becomes malignant.
D. Total colectomy with rectal mucosectomy and endorectal ileal pull trough is technique of choice.
E. Familial adenomatous polyposis is called spare type when polyps are in the hundreds.

Q. 14
Features of Gardner syndrome include all except:

A. Autosomal dominant condition.
B. Associated with familial adenomatous polyposis.
C. Multiple osteoma.
D. Epidermal cyst.
E. Intracranial tumour.

Q. 15
What is false for Peutz–Jeghers syndrome?

A. Polyps most commonly occur in colon.
B. Thirty per cent of patients have signs and symptoms in first year of life.
C. Histologically polyps of Peutz–Jeghers syndrome are hamartoma of muscularis mucosa.
D. Excise polyps more than 5 mm preoperatively and more than 15 mm endoscopically.
E. The risk of cancer is 13 times greater than in the general population.

Q. 16
Intussusception lead point occurs in what percentage of cases?

A. Fewer than 1 percent of cases.
B. 1–2 percent of cases.
C. 2–6 percent of cases.
D. 6–12 percent of cases.
E. 12–20 percent of cases.

Q. 17
About intussusception, which is false?

A. Recurrence is seen in first 48 hours.
B. Success with no operative therapy is widely variable.
C. Young children has more likely pathological lead point especially 3 months to 3 years.
D. Recurrence is more common in children treated by nonoperative ways.
E. Pressure of 80 torr, 100 torr, and then 120 torr (each for 5 minutes), applied in air reduction.

Short Bowel Syndrome

Q. 18
Causes of short bowel syndrome include all except:

   A. Necrotising enterocolitis.
   B. Abdominal wall defect
   C. Multiple atresia.
   D. Sigmoid volvulus.
   E. Congenital short bowel.

Q. 19
Complication of short bowel syndrome include all except:

   A. Constipation.
   B. Fat-soluble vitamins.
   C. gallstones.
   D. Oxalate renal stone.
   E. Lactic acidosis.

Q. 20
Secretion of the following, except one, are the causes of diarrhoea in short-bowel syndrome:

   A. Motilin.
   B. Entero-glucagon.
   C. Cholecystokinin
   D. VIP.
   E. Somatostatin.

Q. 21
Use of the following may be beneficial in short bowel syndrome except:

A. Antibiotics.
B. Parenteral malnutrition.
C. Increases carbohydrate intake.
D. Parental nutrition with high concentration of taurine.
E. Sulphonamide.

Q. 22
The purpose of surgery in short bowel syndrome includes all except:

A. Shortening of intestinal transit.
B. Acceleration of short bowel adaptation.
C. Sequential lengthening of intestine.
D. Restoration of of gut continuity.
E. Correction of partial or complete obstruction.

Q. 23
Which of the following statements is true regarding short bowel syndrome?

A. Adaptation to full enteral feeding occurs in 6 months.
B. Two percent do not develop progressive adaptation.
C. Gallstone occurs in 1–2 percent of cases.
D. Long-term survival rate is 50 percent.
E. In general, patients with 10 cm healthy small bowel beyond the ligamentum trietz and intact ileocecal valve have significant potential for adaptation.

Mesenteric and Omental Cyst

Q. 24
Lymphangioma is different from mesenteric or omental cyst, as it has following features except:

   A. Small lymphatic spaces.
   B. Lymphoid tissues.
   C. Smooth muscles.
   D. Cuboidal or columnar lining of epithelium.
   E. Thin wall.

Q. 25
Intestinal duplication is different from mesenteric cysts on the following bases, except:

   A. Duplication cyst shares common blood supply with adjacent bowel.
   B. Duplication cyst has different mucosal layer from adjacent bowel.
   C. Duplication cyst shares muscular layer from adjacent bowel.
   D. Duplication cyst is macroscopically different from mesenteric cyst.
   E. Duplication cyst is microscopically different from mesenteric cyst.

Q. 26
Which of the following is the most common complication of mesenteric cyst?

   A. Intestinal obstruction.
   B. Haemorrhage.

C. Infection.
D. Obstruction of urinary and biliary tract.
E. Malignancy.

Duplication of Gastrointestinal Tract

Q. 27
What abnormal event occurs during embryonic life that leads to development of duplication list?

    A. Abnormal splitting of notochord.
    B. Abnormal foetal luminal canalization.
    C. Formation of abnormal diverticulum
    D. Squestration of portion of endoderm during development.
    E. All of the above.

Q. 28
Regarding duplication cyst, which of the following is true?

    A. Most of the duplication is thoracoabdominal.
    B. Ectopic gastric mucosa is commonly seen.
    C. Most duplication is solitary.
    D. Most are communicating with bowel.
    E. Ectopic pancreatic tissues are present in 20 per cent of cases.

Q. 29
Regarding duplication cysts, which one is false?

    A. They possess at least one coat of smooth muscle.
    B. They share a common wall with GIT.
    C. They contain some sort of GIT lining.

D. Tubular variety is usually communicating and cystic variety is unusually non-communicating.
E. Tubular variety usually occurs in the stomach and proximal small intestine.

Q. 30
Colonic and rectal duplication cysts seems to be associated with following except:

A. Cloacal exstrophy.
B. Diaphragmatic hernia.
C. Urethral duplication.
D. Spina bifida.
E. Omphalocele.

Q. 31
The followings are different options of treatment of duplication cysts of GIT, except:

A. Resection and end-to-end anastomosis.
B. Injection sclerotherapy.
C. Partial resection with internal drainage of distal end.
D. Partial excision and mucosal stripping.
E. Some duplication cysts may needs Roux-en-Y drainage.

Q. 32
Duodenal duplication has the following features except:

A. Duodenal duplication comprises <6 percent of intestinal duplications.
B. Usually cystic.
C. Communicates with the intestinal lumen.
D. Commonly presents with symptoms of obstruction.

E. Ten to fifteen per cent have ectopic gastric mucosa and can present with bleeding.

Primary Peritonitis

Q. 33
What is false about the primary peritonitis?

A. It is an infectious process of the peritoneal cavity that has intra-abdominal source.
B. The most common organism is Streptococcus pneumonia.
C. An associated common condition is nephrotic syndrome.
D. It may develop in children with splenectomy.
E. It has been in children on long-term steroid treatment.

Acute Appendicitis

Q. 34
Regarding appendicitis in children, which of the following are true?

A. Less chance of mass formation.
B. Less chance of perforation.
C. Laparoscopic appendectomy is a better option in thin patients than obese.
D. Open appendectomy has increased chance of bleeding than laparoscopic.
E. Longer hospital stay in laparoscopic appendectomy.

Q. 35
If on laparotomy appendix is encountered normal, which statement is false?

- A. Appendix should be removed in malrotation.
- B. Appendix should not be removed in Crohn's disease.
- C. Do not remove appendix in patients who are candidate for urological reconstruction.
- D. Do not remove appendix in patient with faecal incontinence.
- E. All of the above are false.

Q. 36
Regarding appendectomy, which one is false?

- A. Lanz incision is a transverse one.
- B. Gridiron incision is an oblique one.
- C. Placement of drain in perforated appendix is optional.
- D. Burring of appendix is an optional procedure.
- E. Duration of post-operative antibiotic in catarrhal appendicitis is 5 days.

Q. 37
The incidence of perforation of appendix in children with appendicitis under 3 years of age is:

- A. 40 percent.
- B. 50 percent.
- C. 60 percent.
- D. 70 percent.
- E. 80 percent.

Intestinal Parasites

Q. 38
The commonest worm that causes intestinal obstruction is:

   A. Tapeworm.
   B. Roundworm.
   C. Flukes.
   D. Hookworm.
   E. Pinworm.

Q. 39
Which of the following vitamin deficiency is caused by Ascaris lumbricoides?

   A. Vitamin A.
   B. Vitamin B1.
   C. Vitamin B2.
   D. Vitamin B6.
   E. Vitamin K.

Q. 40
Which of the following is a characteristic symptom of Loeffler syndrome is caused by Ascaris lumbricoides?

   A. Jaundice.
   B. Abdominal pain
   C. Bloody stool.
   D. Dyspnea.
   E. Dysuria.

Q. 41
Which of the following medications is not used to treat Ascaris lumbricoides worm infestation.

- A. Albendazole.
- B. Mebendazole.
- C. Pyrantel Pamoete.
- D. Penicillin.
- E. Piperazine.

Q. 42
The commonest site for hydatid cyst formation is:

- A. Liver.
- B. Lung.
- C. Brain.
- D. Bone.
- E. Heart.

Q. 43
Sensitivity of indirect haemaglutination test for hydatid cyst is about:

- A. 40 percent.
- B. 50 percent.
- C. 60 percent.
- D. 70 percent.
- E. 80 percent.

Liver Abscess

Q. 44
Regarding liver abscess, which of the following statements is true?

A. Amoebic liver abscess is less common than pyogenic.
B. Left lobe is more commonly involved.
C. Indirect haemaglutination test (IHA) is positive in amoebic liver abscess.
D. Laparotomy and drainage is preferred mode of treatment.
E. Drainage is required if abscess is more than 2 cm.

SECTION 4

UROLOGY A

Urinary Incontinence, Enuresis, and Bladder Reconstructive Procedures

Q. 1
The following are anatomical causes of urinary incontinence, except:

- A. Ectopic ureter.
- B. Posterior urethral valve.
- C. Exstrophy bladder.
- D. Epispadias.
- E. Spinal dysraphism.

Q. 2
The following are functional causes of urinary incontinence except:

- A. Urge syndrome.
- B. Dysfunctional voiding

C. Hinman syndrome.
D. Spinal cord trauma.
E. Giggle incontinence.

Q. 3
Enuresis in children is characterised by all except:

A. It is normal voiding at inappropriate time.
B. When urinary control is expected at 4–6 years of age.
C. It is constant or frequent involuntary passage of urine.
D. It is called primary when the child never been dry.
E. It is called secondary when at least 6 months passed without wetting.

Q. 4
Regarding urinary bladder physiology and maturation, what is not true among the following?

A. Bladder storage is an action of sympathetic from T10, 11, 12 and L1.
B. Newborn bladder capacity is 160 ml.
C. Bladder emptying is an action of parasympathetic S2, S3 and S4.
D. Newborn voids about 20 times a day.
E. Bladder capacity is measured by age in years 2 and up.

Q. 5
In the neuropathic bladder, the following can be expected:

A. Detrusor-sphincter dyssynergia is responsible for failure to emptying the bladder.
B. Inactivity of sphincter leads to incontinence or failure to store.

C. Detrusor overactivity implies small capacity bladder.
D. Detrusor inactivity leads to large-capacity bladder.
E. Overactivity of sphincter mechanism leads to failure of storage of urine.

Q. 6
The following are causes of primary nocturnal enuresis, except:

A. Genetics.
B. Decreased functional bladder capacity.
C. Social factors.
D. Excessive antidiuretic hormones.
E. Food allergies.

Q. 7
Regarding bladder and sphincter reconstructive philosophy, all of the following are true except:

A. To preserve upper urinary tract.
B. Attain socially acceptable continence.
C. High-pressure storage of urine.
D. Maximise child ease of care.
E. To achieve large capacity bladder.

Q. 8
Regarding specific disadvantage of procedure to correct deficient bladder outlet resistance, which of the following is false?

A. The disadvantage of Young-Dees Leadbetter procedure (tabularization of segment of posterior urethra) is that it reduces bladder capacity.

B. The disadvantage of the Croop procedure (use of anterior flap of detrusor) is that it causes difficult catheterization.
C. The disadvantage of facial sling is that it is irreversible.
D. The disadvantage of balloon as artificial sphincter is erosion and infection.
E. The disadvantage of periurethral injection of Teflon is migration of Teflon to lymph nodes, lung, or kidney.

Q. 9
Disadvantages of ileocystoplasty are all except:

A. Alkalosis
B. Mucus production.
C. Infection.
D. Antireflux implantation of ureter is less reliable.
E. Hyperoxalurea and increased incidence of stone formation.

Q. 10
The following factors may trigger stress incontinence except:

A. A sudden cough.
B. Sneezing.
C. Laughing.
D. Heavy lifting.
E. Deep sleep.

Q. 11
Regarding incontinence of urine, which of the following statements is false?

A. Urge incontinence in the presence of urgency.

B. Dysfunctional voiding against a contracted urethral sphincter, resulting in staccato pattern on uroflowmetry.
C. Stress incontinence leakage of urine (usually small amounts) on exertion or with increased intra-abdominal pressure.
D. Giggle incontinence is almost complete voiding occurring during or after laughing with otherwise normal bladder function.
E. All of the above.

Urolithiasis

Q. 12
Of the factors involved in urinary stone formation, which of the following is false?

A. Supersaturation of urinary solutes.
B. Decreases inhibitors of crystallization.
C. Dilution of urinary solutes.
D. Urinary PH.
E. Urinary tract infection.

Q. 13
The following factors predispose urinary stone formation except:

A. Development anomalies of urinary system.
B. Urinary tract infection.
C. Decreased fluid intake.
D. Increased carbohydrate intake.
E. Increased protein intake.

Q. 14
About radio-opaque stones, which entry below is perfect?

A. Calcium oxalate.
B. Calcium phosphate.
C. Cysteine.
D. All of the above.
E. None of the above.

Q. 15
Which of the following metabolic conditions is not associated with urolithiasis?

A. Hyperoxalurea.
B. Hypecalciurea.
C. Hypercitrateurea.
D. Cysteineurea.
E. Xanthineurea

Q. 16
About detection of radiolucent stones, which of the following entries below is perfect?

A. By intravenous urography.
B. By ultrasound.
C. By CT scan.
D. By all of the above.
E. By none of the above.

Q. 17
In urolithiasis management, which of the following is not true?

A. ESWL (Extra-corporeal shock wave lithotripsy) is good for large/staghorn stones.
B. ESWL is suitable for stones in lower ureter in females.
C. Open surgery is suitable when there are big stones and distal obstruction.
D. Percutaneous nephrolithotomy procedure can be combined with ESWL.
E. Electrohydraulic methods can be used in cystolithopaxy and percutaneous nephrolithotomy.

Q. 18
Which stone is formed when urease-producing organisms alkalinise the urine?

A. Xanthine.
B. Struvite.
C. Uric acid.
D. Cysteine.
E. Calcium oxalate.

Q. 19
Prominent features of metabolic stones are all of the following except:

A. Age less than 3 years.
B. Stone in lower urinary tract.
C. Multiple stones.
D. Nephrocalcinosis.
E. Positive family history.

Q. 20
For extracorporeal shockwave lithotripsy (ESWL), all of the following statements are true except:

A. Plenty of oral liquid is advised after ESWL.
B. Antibiotics and analgesics may be required.
C. X-rays are advised after 7–10 days.
D. Repeat sessions of ESWL may be required not earlier than 7–10 days.
E. ESWL is suitable for stones larger than 2.5 cm.

Q. 21
Colour of cysteine stones is:

A. Black.
B. White.
C. Green.
D. Pink.
E. Brown.

Vesicoureteric Reflux

Q. 22
Which of the following is not a cause of vesicoureteric reflux?

A. Long intravesical submucosal tunnel.
B. Per ureteric diverticulum.
C. Prune belly syndrome.
D. Ureterocele.
E. Posterior urethral valve.

Q. 23
The international classification of vesicoureteric reflux for patients with dilated calyces but fornics are sharp, stands for which grade of reflux.

A. Grade I.
B. Grade II.
C. Grade III.
D. Grade IV.
E. Grade V.

Q. 24
The indications for surgical ureteric re-implantation include all of the below except:

A. Repeated breakthrough urinary tract infection (UTI) during antibiotic prophylactic.
B. Anatomical abnormality of vesicoureteric junction.
C. Persistent reflux in an adolescence that has not resolved.
D. Vesicoureteric reflux in an association with ureteric obstruction.
E. Grade II reflux.

Q. 25
For surgical procedure of vesicoureteric reimplantation, which of the following is false?

A. New hiatus is created in extravesical approach.
B. New hiatus is created through intravesical approach.
C. Detrusor is approximated in extravesical approach.
D. Ureter is passed through tunnel in intravesical approach.
E. All of the above are false.

Q. 26
In ureteric reimplantation, the ratio between tunnel length and ureteric diameter should be:

A. 2:1
B. 2:2
C. 5:3
D. 5:1
E. 6:3

Q. 27
In STING (sub-ureteric transurethral injection), which of the following is not true?

A. DEFLU is the material used for injection.
B. PTFE (Polytetrafluoroethylene) can also be used.
C. Injection is given at the 12 o'clock position at the affected ureteric orifice.
D. The needle is advanced in 4–5 mm in lamina propria.
E. Most refluxing ureter requires less than 0.3 ml of biologically inert material.

Q. 28
Regarding vesicoureteric reflux, which of the following statements is not false?

A. Incidence in normal population is about 5 perent.
B. Proteus is the most common organism seen in urine culture.
C. Renal scarring is noted in fewer than 10 per cent of cases.
D. Cessation of vesicoureteric reflux after one STING is about 50 percent.

E. There is no difficulty if secondary surgery is needed after STING procedure.

Q. 29
In international classification of vesicoureteral reflux, which grade you will label if partial filling with undilated ureter?

A. Grade I.
B. Grade II.
C. Grade III.
D. Grade IV.
E. Grade IV.

Partial Nephrectomy

Q. 30
Which of the following is not true about open partial nephrectomy?

A. Ureteric duplication with non-functioning upper pole is a common indication.
B. Renal segment to be removed is difficult to identify.
C. Mattress sutures can be placed to approximate the ages of renal parenchyma.
D. The ureter is removed as low as possible.
E. Ischaemia to remnant kidney is due to traction spasm or traction injury to renal vessels.

Ureteric Duplication, Ectopic Ureter, and Ureterocele

Q. 31
Regarding the ectopic ureter, which of the following is not true?

A. If a second ureteric bud arises in more caudal than normal location, the ureter is incorporated into the developing ureter in a more proximal location.
B. In males, the ectopic ureter enters the genitoureteric tract above the external urethral sphincter.
C. Urinary incontinence is less often seen in females with ectopic ureter than in males.
D. Ectopic ureter is more common in female.
E. About 20 percent are bilateral.

Q. 32
Which is true in relation to ectopic ureter?

A. Dilated upper moiety is difficult to identify by ultrasound.
B. Methylene blue test should not be used to see leakage.
C. Epididymitis and prostatitis is not the way of presentation.
D. If kidney function is good, ureteric reimplantation in single system or ureteropyloplasty or double-barrel reimplantation for duplex system is justified.
E. Continent diversion is needed in most cases.

Q. 33
Regarding ureterocele, which of the following is not true?

A. It is associated with single or double ureter.
B. In duplex kidney, it occurs generally as dilatation of terminal part of upper pole of ureter.
C. When it is intravesical, it is called orthotopic.
D. Sphinteric is a type of ectopic ureterocele.
E. All of the above are false.

Q. 34
Which of the following statements is true in ureterocele?

    A. Stenotic variety is entirely contained within the bladder.
    B. Most ureterocele with single ureter are ectopic.
    C. Most ureterocele with duplex system are orthotopic.
    D. Ultrasound shows "cobra-head" appearance.
    E. Ureterocele with reimplantation is the first choice of procedure.

Q. 35
Regarding ureteric duplication, which one is false?

    A. Two ureteric buds arising from mesonephric duct usually lead to complete duplication with no abnormality.
    B. Single ureteric bud arising but bifurcating shortly leads to duplication with duplex kidney and ectopic ureter.
    C. In duplex system, upper pole ureter is anterior to lower pole ureter in intravesical course.
    D. In duplex system, upper pole ureter is posterior to lower pole ureter in intramural tunnel.
    E. All of the above are false.

Mega Ureter and Prune-Belly Syndrome

Q. 36
Which of the following related to megaureter is false?

    A. It is caused by obstruction, vesicoureteric reflux, or prune-belly syndrome.
    B. Principle of surgery tapering and reimplantation in bladder with tension, angulation and ischaemia.

C. In preimplantation, ratio of tunnel length to diameter of ureteric orifice must be 5:1.
D. Repair of upper ureter is needed in most cases.
E. Reflux and obstruction are main complications of surgery.

Q. 37
In prune-belly syndrome, which of the following statements is false?

A. There is hyperdynamic segment of lower ureter.
B. Ureter contains more collagen and less fibre tissues.
C. The triad includes deficiency of abdominal wall musculature, hydroureteronephrossis, and cryptorchidism.
D. Almost all patients are male.
E. All of the above.

Q. 38
Regarding prune-belly syndrome, which statement is true?

A. The treatment is controversial.
B. Watchful waiting is an option.
C. For abdominal wall partial, resection and tailoring is an option.
D. Fowler-Stephens technique can be is used for orchidopexy.
E. All of the above.

Diversion and Undiversion

Q. 39
Which of the following is not a variety of continent urinary diversion?

   A. Kock pouch.
   B. Indiana pouch.
   C. Mainz pouch.
   D. Mitrofanoff stoma.
   E. End ureterostomy.

Posterior Urethral Valve

Q. 40
Which of the following is true related to posterior urethral valve?

   A. Type I is straight oriented diaphragm.
   B. Type II is most common.
   C. It inhibits detrusor atrophy.
   D. Proximal urethra is shortened and dilated.
   E. Bladder neck is secondarily narrowed.

Q. 41
Features of posterior urethral valve include all except:

   A. Thin-walled bladder on in-utero ultrasound.
   B. Infant with thin stream.
   C. Retention of urine.
   D. Incontinence of urine.
   E. Hypertension.

Q. 42
Investigations of posterior urethral valve can show all except:

A. Dilatation of anterior urethra.
B. Thick-walled bladder.
C. High post voiding residual.
D. Hydroureteronephrosis.
E. Vesicoureteric reflux.

Q. 43
Management of posterior urethral valve include all except:

A. Initial vesicostomy is a better option in premature babies.
B. Initial valve ablation is a better option than vesicostomy in unstable patients.
C. Valve is ablated in the 5, 7 and 12 o'clock positions.
D. After valve ablation, MCUG is done after 3 months.
E. The child is followed till puberty.

Q. 44
Perfect answer related to complications of posterior urethral valve is:

A. Hydroureter.
B. Renal failure.
C. Hypertension.
D. All of the above.
E. None of the above.

Q. 45
The common anatomical location of the posterior urethral valve is:

- A. Proximal to prostatic urethra.
- B. Distal to verumontanum.
- C. Distal to bulbar urethra.
- D. In penile urethra.
- E. At glandular urethra.

Q. 46
Regarding complications of the posterior urethral valve, which of the following is not true?

- A. Urine culture is positive in most cases.
- B. Chronic renal failure is an important cause of mortality.
- C. Retrograde ejaculation is one of the complications.
- D. Urodynamic abnormalities seen in 20 percent of cases.
- E. Bladder dysfunction manifests as incontinence of urine.

Q. 47
Voiding cystourethrogram (VCUG) shows the specific sign in posterior urethral valve is:

- A. Sandwich sign.
- B. Doughnut sign.
- C. String sign.
- D. Keyhole sign.
- E. Murphy sign.

Q. 48
The most common effect of back pressure in the posterior urethral valve is:

A. Bladder diverticulum.
B. Vesicoureteric reflux.
C. Hydronephrosis.
D. All of the above.
E. None of the above.

Q. 49
Which of the following investigations best shows scarring of the kidney?

A. DTPA.
B. DMSA.
C. MAG3.
D. All of the above.
E. None of the above

SECTION 5

UROLOGY B

Renal Agenesis, Dysplasia and Cystic Disease, Renal Fusion, and Ectopia

Q. 1
Polycystic kidney shows the following features except:

A. Many cysts in both kidneys
B. No continuity between glomeruli and calyces
C. Congenital variety is autosomal recessive
D. Adult variety is autosomal dominant
E. No renal dysplasia

Q. 2
Regarding anomalies related to abnormal ascent of the kidney (ectopic kidney), which of the following statements is true?

A. Thoracic ectopic kidney is the most common.
B. Pelvic ectopic kidney is a rare variety.
C. Iliac variety is fixed below the crest of the ileum.

D. Lumbar variety is below the level of L2 and L3.
E. Lumbar and iliac ectopic kidney are the same thing.

Q. 3
Horseshoe kidney shows the following features except:

A. It is the most common fusion defect.
B. In 95 per cent of cases, the upper poles of the kidney are joined.
C. The bridge of tissues between two kidneys can be either normal, dysplastic or fibrous tissue.
D. It is postulated that inferior mesenteric artery obstructs the isthmus and prevents ascent.
E. Correction of ureteropelvic junction obstruction is the most frequent indication for surgical intervention.

Pelviureteric Junction Obstruction

Q. 4
Features of pelviureteric junction (PUJ) obstruction include all of the following except:

A. Dilated pelvis after 18 weeks of gestation.
B. Low sodium in foetal bladder urine.
C. Absence of dilated ureter.
D. Delayed passage of contrast through PUJ.
E. Renal scarring.

Q. 5
Which of the following is not an appropriate statement for management of PUJ obstruction?

A. Conservative management is justified in the asymptomatic child.
B. Temporary diversion of urine (percutaneous nephrostomy) is indicated in infants with severe unilateral dilatation.
C. Surgical treatment is indicated in declining function of dilated kidney.
D. In foetus, urinary diversion is indicated in unilateral dilated pelvis.
E. In foetus, pelviamnoitic shunt is the procedure of choice.

Q. 6
Which of the following is not complication of pyeloplasty for PUJ obstruction?

A. Recurrent stenosis.
B. Renal shutdown.
C. Metabolic alkalosis.
D. Hypertension.
E. Stone formation.

Q. 7
Regarding PUJ obstruction, which statement is false?

A. External compression and blockage by aberrant vessels and adhesive band occurs in most of cases.
B. Incidence is 1:1000.
C. Abdominal mass, pain, and recurrent UTI are the presenting features.

D. Extra-peritoneal or trans-peritoneal approach can be used.
E. Ureter is speculated in Anderson-Hynes procedure.

Q. 8
Regarding antenatal hydronephrosis, which of the following statements is true?

A. Antenatal hydronephrosis is diagnosed as early as second trimester of pregnancy.
B. Posterior urethral valve may be the cause of blockage in females.
C. Most cases are followed by CT scan during pregnancy.
D. Severe obstruction in both kidneys leads to oligohydramnios.
E. PUJ and vesicoureteric junction are not causes of antenatal hydronephrosis.

Exstrophy Bladder

Q. 9
Regarding embryology of exstrophy bladder, which of the following is false?

A. Abnormal underdevelopment of cloacal membrane.
B. Prevention of migration of mesenchymal tissue.
C. Inappropriate development of lower abdominal wall and pubis.
D. Problem in position and timing of rupture of anterior portion of cloacal membrane.
E. Fifty per cent are of the classical variety.

Q. 10
Findings in exstrophy bladder include all except:

A. Everted posterior bladder wall of varying size.
B. Early union of symphysis pubis.
C. Ureteric orifice may be obvious.
D. Mucosa may be normal or it may be fibrotic rigid.
E. Direct or indirect inguinal hernia.

Q. 11
Genitourinary defects in exstrophy bladder include all except:

A. There are undescended testes, which eventually reside without need for orchidopexy in most cases.
B. Distance between umbilicus and anus is foreshortened.
C. Anus is posteriorly placed.
D. Anal sphincter mechanism is displaced anteriorly.
E. Prepuce is on ventral aspect of penis.

Q. 12
Genital defects in females with exstrophy bladder include all except:

A. Clitoris is characteristically bifid with divergence of labia.
B. Urethra and vagina are short.
C. Vaginal orifice is almost always displaced anteriorly.
D. Vagina is often dilated.
E. There is deficient pelvis floor.

Q. 13
Variants of exstrophy bladder include all except:

A. Covered exstrophy.
B. Duplicate exstrophy.
C. Superior vesical fissure.
D. Pseudoexstrophy.
E. Exomphalos.

Q. 14
Management of exstrophy of bladder includes all except:

A. Primary closure at birth.
B. Epispadias repair at one year in males.
C. Continent reconstruction at two years of age.
D. Bladder augmentation at 4 years in males.
E. Osteotomy at birth, if needed.

Hypospadias

Q. 15
Regarding embryology of external genitalia, which of the following is true?

A. External genitalia is masculinised by Mullerian inhibiting substance.
B. Embryonic male urethra has two separate segments.
C. Midline fusion of labioscrotal fold forms perineal membrane.
D. Glanular urethra is formed by mesodermal intrusion at the tip of glans.
E. Mesenchyme in urethral fold forms corpus spongiosum.

Q. 16
Regarding classification of hypospadias, which of the following is false?

   A. Anterior hypospadias is commonest variety because this is the last step in the formation of complete urethra.
   B. Middle hypospadias includes distal penile, mid-shaft and proximal penile variety.
   C. Penoscrotal hypospadias is a variety of anterior hypospadias.
   D. Middle variety accounts about 30 percent of hypospadias.
   E. Posterior hypospadias is least common.

Q. 17
Element of hypospadias anomaly include all except:

   A. Meatal dystopia.
   B. Dermal defect.
   C. Penile curvature.
   D. Peyronie's disease.
   E. Penoscrotal transposition and bifid scrotum.

Q. 18
What do you do in repair of hypospadias.

   A. Orthoplasty (straightening).
   B. Urethroplasty, glanuloplasty and meatoplasty.
   C. Skin cover.
   D. All of the above
   E. None of above.

Q. 19
Regarding repair of hypospadias, all are false except:

A. Meatal advancement and glanuloplasty (MAGPI) is a procedure for midpenile hypospadias.
B. In Mathieu repair, flap of tissue is raised from distal to meatus.
C. In Onlay Island flap urethroplasty, urethral plate is removed.
D. In Mustarde procedure, tunnel is made under the urethral plate.
E. Intraoperative, to check whether penis is straight or not, penis is stretched repeatedly.

Cloacal Exstrophy

Q. 20
Regarding cloacal exstrophy, which of the following is false?

A. It is caused by rupture of cloacal membrane after anorectal septum has completely descended.
B. Males are more commonly affected than females.
C. The hemibladder is most commonly situated on either side of centrally situated on either side of centrally placed atrophied strip of intestine (usually caecum).
D. Uterus or vagina may be duplicated.
E. The incidence of associated anomalies is much higher than in classical bladder exstrophy.

Q. 21
Regarding treatment of cloacal exstrophy, all are true except:

A. It is managed in multidisciplinary fashion.

B. Sex assignment and rapid karyotyping is needed.
C. Karyotype male is kept as male.
D. Survival is 90 percent.
E. Cause of death is prematurity, renal agenesis, and associated anomalies.

Q. 22
For cloacal exstrophy, none of the following is done at birth except:

A. Bladder neck reconstruction.
B. Urethral preimplantation.
C. Mitrofanoff procedure.
D. Repair of omphalocele.
E. Gastric augmentation.

Ambiguous Genitalia

Q. 23
Features of female pseudohermaphrodite include all except:

A. Karyotype 46XX (chromatin positive).
B. Electrolyte shows high potassium and low sodium.
C. High androgen.
D. High 17-hydro-oxyprogestrone.
E. Asymmetrical gonads.

Q. 24
Features of mixed gonadal dysgenesis include all except:

A. Asymmetry of gonads.
B. Urogenital sinus defect.
C. Clitoral hypertrophy.

D. Karyotype 46XX.
E. Low testosterone.

Q. 25
When a true hermaphrodite is raised as female, the following management is required except:

A. Clitoral recession.
B. Vaginal exteriorization.
C. Removal of Mullerian structures.
D. Labioscrotal reduction.
E. Preserve normal ovary.

Q. 26
Regarding ambiguous genitalia, which of the following is false?

A. Mixed gonadal dysgenesis is the most common chromosomal abnormality.
B. Pure gonadal dysgenesis may have defective Y chromosomes.
C. Mixed gonadal dysgenesis may undergo neoplastic transformation (gonadoblastoma or seminoma).
D. When ovarian and testicular tissues coexist in same gonads, ovarian tissues are always central and testicular tissues are polar.
E. Pure gonadal dysgenesis does not undergo neoplastic transformation.

Q. 27
The most common deficiency in congenital adrenal hyperplasia is:

A. 11 hydroxylase.

B. 21 hydroxylase.
C. 31 hydroxylase.
D. 11 dehydroxylase.
E. 21 dehydroxylase.

Testicular Torsion

Q. 28
Regarding features of testicular torsion, all of the following are true except:

A. Extravaginal torsion is more common.
B. Peak age is 13–16 years.
C. Torsion of appendix testes is more common than true torsion of testes.
D. Sudden pain, swelling, and redness of scrotum is best treated as torsion of testes.
E. Doppler ultrasound is less helpful in infants.

Q. 29
Regarding torsion of testes, which one is false?

A. Immediate operative exploration is required.
B. Testes should be untwisted and assessed for viability.
C. Do orchiectomy of ischaemic gonad in child above 10 years in case of dead testes.
D. In adolescents with recurrent testicular pain, bilateral orchidopexy is justified.
E. Idiopathic scrotal oedema is not a differential diagnosis.

Undescended Testes

Q. 30
Regarding embryology of descend of testes, all are false except:

A. Gubernaculum is attached at upper pole of testes.
B. Processus vaginalis grows cranially into the gubernaculum.
C. Process of descend accomplished by 35 weeks.
D. Androgen control regression of gubernaculum.
E. Mullerian inhibiting substance causes regression of gubernaculum.

Q. 31
Low abdominal pressure is the cause of undescended testes in all of the following except:

A. Omphalocele.
B. Gastroschisis.
C. Prune Belly syndrome.
D. Microcephaly.
E. Neural tube defect.

Q. 32
Which of the following is not true of ectopic testes?

A. Femoral.
B. Perineal.
C. Pubopenile.
D. Transverse ectopia (In contralateral hemiscrotum).
E. Intra-abdominal.

Q. 33
In retractile testes, which statement is true?

A. Dartos muscle contraction causes retraction of testes.
B. Ileoinguinal nerve is responsible.
C. Careful follow-up is required.
D. This is a variety of undescended testes.
E. Surgery is never required.

Q. 34
Complications of undescended testes include all the below except:

A. Affected endocrine function of Sertoli and Lydig cell.
B. Fall in the number of germ cells.
C. Decrease in fertility.
D. Increased incidence of testicular trauma.
E. Ecreased incidence of torsion of testes.

Q. 35
In the management of undescended testes, which of the following is false?

A. Diagnosis is usually clinical.
B. Beta HCG and LHRH has high success rate.
C. Orchidopexy is done in 6–12 months.
D. Orchiectomy, if testes is small and dysgenetic.
E. Intra-abdominal testes has poor prognosis.

Q. 36
Regarding malignancy in undescended testes, all are true except:

A. Relative risk in undescended testes is 5–10 times.
B. There is no conclusion that orchiectomy reduces the risk of malignancy.
C. Placement of testes in scrotum in scrotum facilitates early diagnosis of malignancy, if it occurs.
D. Most testicular tumours in childhood occur in undescended testes.
E. The most common age range for cancer to occur in an undescended testes is 20–40 years.

SECTION 6

THORACIC SURGERY

Congenital Diaphragmatic Hernia

Q. 1
Regarding development of the diaphragm, which of the following is correct.

- A. Central tendon develops from pleuroperitoneal membrane.
- B. Dorsolateral part develops from pleuroperitoneal membrane.
- C. Dorsal crura develops from thoracic intercostal muscle.
- D. Muscular part develops from septum transversum.
- E. None of the above.

Q. 2
Commonest cause of development of Bochdalek hernia is weakness in:

- A. Central tendon.
- B. Dorsolateral part.

C. Dorsal crura.
D. Muscular part.
E. None of the above.

Q. 3
Which one is the commonest varieties of congenital hernia?

A. Hiatus hernia.
B. Bochdalek hernia.
C. Morgagni hernia.
D. Umbilical hernia.
E. Epigastric hernia.

Q. 4
Herniation of abdominal viscera occurs at which age of foetal life to develop diaphragmatic hernia.

A. 7–8 weeks.
B. 9–10 weeks.
C. 11–12 weeks.
D. 13 to 14 weeks.
E. 15 to 16 weeks.

Q. 5
Regarding symptoms of diaphragmatic hernia, the perfect answer is:

A. Pulmonary hypertension.
B. Pulmonary hypoplasia.
C. Size of defect.
D. A and B are correct.
E. B and C are correct.

Q. 6
At birth, which of the following is not a feature of congenital diaphragmatic hernia?

   A. Respiratory distress.
   B. Distended abdomen.
   C. Funnel chest.
   D. Gasping.
   E. Cyanosis.

Q. 7
Fluoroscopy helps to differentiate Bochdalek hernia from which of the following conditions?

   A. Morgagni hernia.
   B. Eventration of diaphragm.
   C. Hiatus hernia.
   D. Congenital cystic disease of lung.
   E. Primary agenesis of lung.

Q. 8
Anatomical factors of prognosis of congenital diaphragmatic hernia include all except:

   A. Presence of oligohydramnios.
   B. Associated significant anomaly.
   C. Position of the stomach in chest.
   D. Right-sided defects.
   E. Cardiac wall thickness.

Q. 9
Procedure for repair of diaphragmatic hernia includes all except:

A. Primary repair of non-absorbable suture.
B. Diaphragm sutured to body wall.
C. Plication of diaphragm.
D. Use of prosthetic material to repair of defect.
E. Use of prerenal fascia.

Q. 10

Features and management of eventration of diaphragm caused by phrenic nerve injury is different from congenital variety in the following ways, except:

A. Has normal distribution of muscle.
B. Observe for 2–4 weeks for return of function of diaphragm.
C. Portion of diaphragm not needs to be excised at the time of repair.
D. For right-sided Eventration, thoracic approach is preferred.
E. Has normal central tendinous area.

Q. 11

What percentage of diaphragmatic hernias are left-sided?

A. 15 percent.
B. 35 percent.
C. 55 percent.
D. 75 percent
E. 95 percent.

Q. 12
Morgagni hernia represents what percentage of congenital diaphragmatic hernia?

   A. 1–3 percent of cases.
   B. 2–5 percent of cases.
   C. 5–8 percent of cases.
   D. 8–10 percent of cases.
   E. 10–15 percent of cases.

Q. 13
The most common chromosomal abnormality identified in congenital diaphragmatic hernia, when diagnosed in utero, is:

   A. Trisomy 13.
   B. Trisomy 18.
   C. Trisomy 21.
   D. Deletion of short arm of chromosome number 9.
   E. Deletion of long arm of chromosome number 18.

Q. 14
Long-term problems after repair of diaphragmatic hernia include all except:

   A. Gastroesophageal reflux.
   B. Failure to thrive.
   C. Hyperinflation of lung.
   D. Respiratory insufficiency.
   E. Recurrence.

Q. 15
X-ray chest findings in congenital diaphragmatic hernia include all except:

A. Loops of intestine.
B. Gastric bubble.
C. Nasogastric tube position in chest.
D. Shifting of mediastinum to same side.
E. Invisible complete dome of diaphragm.

Oesophageal Atresia

Q. 16
Gastroesophageal reflux is a complication of oesophageal atresia repair; which of the following procedures do you do for its correction.

A. Oesophageal dilatation.
B. Resection and anastomosis.
C. Oesophageal replacement.
D. Fundoplication.
E. Aortopexy.

Q. 17
For VACTERAL association, all of the following statements are false except:

A. V stands for vaginal atresia.
B. A stands for arterial lesion.
C. C stands for coronary lesion.
D. T stands for thoracic wall anomaly.
E. R stands for renal anomaly.

Q. 18
In CHARGE association, all of the following are true except:

A. C stands for coloboma.
B. H stands for heart defect.
C. A stands for atresia choanea.
D. R stands for developmental retardation.
E. E stands for Oesophageal atresia.

Q. 19
Regarding oesophageal atresia, which of the following is false?

A. Foetal ultrasound shows upper oesophageal pouch, filling, and emptying.
B. If foetal ultrasound is unable to detect stomach, this indicates atresia without fistula.
C. Failure to advance nasogastric tube 10 cm beyond mouth or nose.
D. Cyanotic episode, frothing, and respiratory distress are all common symptoms.
E. Choice of operation is oesophagostomy and gastrostomy when patient is fit.

Q. 20
Regarding thoracotomy for oesophageal atresia, which of the following is false?

A. Ligation and division of azygos vein.
B. Identification and preservation of recurrent laryngeal nerve.
C. Identification and mobilisation of lower pouch and fistula.

D. Single-layer anastomosis.
E. Chest drain is optional.

Q. 21
Indication of cervical oesophagostomy includes all except:

A. Short gap oesophageal atresia.
B. When attempt of primary anastomosis of oesophagus fails.
C. Disruption of primary anastomosis.
D. Extensive stricture of oesophagus after caustic ingestion.
E. Foreign body perforation of oesophagus.

Q. 22
Regarding procedure of cervical oesophagostomy, which one is correct?

A. Right side preferred.
B. Incision 1 cm above and parallel to lateral third of clavicle.
C. Ligation and division of external jugular vein.
D. Retract carotid artery, internal jugular vein, and vagus nerve medially.
E. Identify and divide recurrent laryngeal nerve.

Q. 23
Regarding H-type congenital tracheoesophageal fistula, which of the following is false?

A. Tube oesophagogram is in supine position.
B. Bronchoscopy and oesophagoscopy can confirm the diagnosis.

C. Cervical approach is more commonly used for ligation and division.
D. Inferior thyroid artery and middle thyroid vein is ligated and divided.
E. Preserve recurrent laryngeal nerve.

Q. 24
Regarding oesophageal rupture, which of the following is false?

A. Boerhaave syndrome refers to oesophageal rupture secondary to forceful vomiting and retching.
B. In neonates, left-sided pneumothorax is more common.
C. Surgical empyema may be present.
D. Oesophagoscopy offers no diagnostic advantage.
E. Decision depends upon site of perforation.

Q. 25
Regarding complications of oesophageal atresia, the following statements are true except:

A. There is direct relationship between post-operative leakage and the gap between two ends of oesophagus.
B. Leakage is noted in 10–20 percent of cases.
C. All those who develop dysphagia require surgery.
D. Incidence of gastroesophageal reflux is about 50 percent.
E. Incidence of scoliosis increases with second thoracotomy.

Q. 26
In oesophageal atresia, a tube meets atretic pouch of oesophagus usually at what distance from lip or nostril?

A. 4–6 cm.
B. 8–12 cm.

C. 14–18 cm.
D. 20 cm.
E. More than 20 cm.

Q. 27
The most common type of oesophageal atresia is:

A. Oesophageal atresia with proximal tracheoesophageal fistula.
B. Oesophageal atresia with distal tracheoesophageal fistula.
C. Oesophageal atresia with fistula to both pouches.
D. H-type fistula (no atresia).
E. Isolated atresia (no fistula).

Q. 28
About associated anomalies in oesophageal atresia, all are true except:

A. Overall associated anomalies are 50–70 percent.
B. Cardiovascular anomalies are 29–35 percent.
C. Gastrointestinal anomalies are 10 percent.
D. Genitourinary anomalies are found in 20 percent cases.
E. Neurological defect has been seen in 10 percent cases.

Q. 29
Incidence of anastomotic leak noted in oesophageal atresia with tracheoesophageal atresia repair is:

A. 5–10 percent of cases.
B. 10–20 percent cases.
C. 20–30 percent cases.

D. 30–40 percent cases.
E. 40–50 percent cases.

Q. 30
Recurrent tracheoesophageal fistula is noted in:

A. less than 1 per cent cases.
B. 1–2 percent cases.
C. 2–5 percent cases.
D. 5–8 percent cases.
E. 8–10 percent cases.

Q. 31
H-type variety of congenital tracheoesophageal fistula is usually repaired by which of the following incision?

A. Right cervical incision.
B. Right thoracic incision
C. Midline abdominal incision.
D. All are useful.
E. None of the above.

Q. 32
Isolated oesophageal atresia comprises what percentage of oesophageal atresia?

A. 2–4 percent.
B. 6–8 percent.
C. 10–12 percent.
D. 14–16 percent.
E. 18–20 percent.

Aortopexy

Q. 33
Regarding aortopexy, which of the following is false?

A. Right anterior thoracotomy is preferred.
B. Incision at the level of third rib.
C. Internal memory vessels at the medial end of the incision is divided.
D. Lobe of thymus is divided with care of to preserve phrenic nerve.
E. Adventitia of aorta and pericardium is sutured with the posterior surface of sternum.

Oesophageal Replacement

Q. 34
About indication of oesophageal replacement with colon, which one of the following is the best answer?

A. Oesophageal atresia with inadequate length for primary anastomosis.
B. Stricture that is too long for resection and anastomosis.
C. Extensive Barrett's oesophagus in the distal oesophagus.
D. All of the above are correct.
E. None of the above are correct.

Q. 35
The best answer among following for oesophageal replacement with colon is:

A. Right colon is used.
B. Transverse colon is used.

C. Left colon is used.
D. Any of above is used.
E. None of the above is used.

Q. 36
The preferred approach for oesophageal replacement with colon is:

A. Right thoracotomy.
B. Left thoracotomy.
C. Midline sternotomy.
D. All of the above.
E. None of the above.

Caustic Ingestion

Q. 37
Which of the following is considered alkali, causing caustic strictures of oesophagus?

A. Hydrochloric acid.
B. Sodium hydro-oxide.
C. Ammonium hydro-oxide.
D. Sodium hypochlorite.
E. Sodium polyphosphate.

Q. 38
Regarding Injury after caustic ingestion, all of the following statements are correct except:

A. Acid causes liquefactive necrosis.
B. Oesophagus is primarily damaged at area of holdup.
C. Perforation of oesophagus may occur.

D. Fibrosis and shortening may lead to shortening of oesophagus.
E. Aortoesophageal fistula may develop.

Q. 39
Regarding caustic ingestion and oesophagus, all of the following are true except:

A. Damage is directly related to the concentration of a caustic substance.
B. In case of alkali ingestion, induction of vomiting is contraindicated.
C. Fiberoptic endoscopy is indicated after 48 hours.
D. Contrast oesophagogram is done at 2 weeks.
E. If fever, sepsis and upper abdominal signs are present, perforation may have occurred.

Q. 40
Regarding endoscopic grading of oesophageal injury after caustic ingestion, which statement is true?

A. Grade I is blister formation and superficial ulcer.
B. Grade IIa is a deep discrete or circumferential ulcer.
C. Grade IIb is small scattered area of necrosis.
D. Grade IIIa is extensive necrosis.
E. All of the above are false.

Q. 41
Poor prognostic factor in stricture of oesophagus following caustic ingestion include all except:

A. Delayed presentation.
B. Extensive grade III injury.

C. Delayed fibrotic stricture that cracks on dilatation.
D. Stricture longer than 2 cm.
E. Inadequate lumen patency despite if repeated dilatation over 9–12 months.

Gastroesophageal Reflux

Q. 42
Closing mechanism for lower oesophageal sphincter, those acts as antireflux barrier include all except:

A. Pinch cock action of sling-shaped orifice formed by right crus of diaphragm.
B. Angle of His that is an acute angle between fundus of stomach and oesophagus.
C. Gastric contraction.
D. Mucosal rosette, convoluted fold of mucosa at gastroesophageal junction.
E. High pressure zone at oesophagus and gastric cardia.

Q. 43
Regarding intraabdominal length of oesophagus and gastroesophageal reflux, which of the following is false?

A. Intraabdominal length of oesophagus has a vital role in presenting reflux.
B. Intraabdominal length more than 5 cm is sufficient in infants to prevent reflux.
C. Intraabdominal length of 1 cm is sufficient.
D. After birth pars abdominals grows faster than pars thoracalis, so it helps in controlling reflux.

E. The greater the abdominal length more the vale becomes, when the intraabdominal pressure increases the oesophagus response as soft tube and collapse.

Q. 44
Consequences of gastroesophageal reflux include all except:

A. Oesophagitis.
B. Oesophageal stricture.
C. Barrett's syndrome.
D. Squamous cell carcinoma of oesophagus.
E. Pneumonia.

Q. 45
Regarding the role of investigation in gastroesophageal reflux, all of the following are false except:

A. In pH monitoring, the oesophagus is alternatively perfused with 0.1N Hcl and saline solution through the nasogastric tube.
B. The Bernstein test, also demonstrated by pulmonary aspiration.
C. Oesophageal manometry demonstrates impaired peristalsis.
D. Gastroesophageal scintigraphy is not helpful because of the high dose of radiation.
E. Endoscopy has a role in controlled gastroesophageal reflux.

Q. 46
Non-operative treatment in gastroesophageal reflux includes all of the following except:

A. Trendelenburg position.
B. Prokinetic drug.
C. Antacids.
D. H2 receptor blocker.
E. Proton pump inhibitor.

Q. 47
Indication for surgical treatment in gastroesophageal reflux include all except:

A. Oesophagitis with development of stricture.
B. Persistent chronic pulmonary disease.
C. Failure of medical treatment
D. Obesity.
E. Secondary causes of gastroesophageal reflux.

Q. 48
Regarding surgery for gastroesophageal reflux, which of the following statements is true?

A. Nissan fundoplication is 180-degree anterior wrap of fundus with intraabdominal oesophagus.
B. Sutures are placed through full thickness, including mucosa.
C. Thal-Ashcraft is a 360-degree complete wrap of fundus of stomach with oesophagus.
D. Restoration of angle of His in Thal-Ashcraft.
E. Fundus of stomach is opened and unfolded in Nissan procedure.

Thoracic Cavity

Q. 49
Indication of pulmonary resection in tuberculosis includes all of the following except:

A. An open cavity that persists after 6 months of combined drug therapy.
B. The inadequate pulmonary reserve.
C. Irreversible destructive lesion.
D. An unexpandable lobe with encapsulating empyema.
E. Recurrent persistent haemorrhage.

Q. 50
Regarding actinomycosis, which of the following is false?

A. It causes lymphadenitis.
B. It causes lung abscess formation.
C. It causes sinus formation.
D. Sulphur granules are pathognomonic.
E. Amphotericin B is the treatment.

Q. 51
Regarding bronchiectasis, which of the following is true?

A. It is an abnormal constriction of bronchi and bronchiole.
B. Asthma is the cause.
C. X-rays show increased bronchovesicular marking.
D. Mostly occurs in apical segment.
E. Pulmonary resection is commonly required.

Q. 52
What is the most common cause of empyema thorax?

A. Trauma.
B. Intrathoracic oesophageal perforation.
C. Surgery on chest.
D. Pneumonia.
E. Bronchiectasis.

Q. 53
Regarding chylothrax in children, which of the following is false?

A. Chylothrax in new-born may be spontaneous.
B. Lymphoma is one of the causes of chylothrax.
C. Persistent central venous catheter is a rare cause.
D. Leakage in lower part of thoracic duct causes left-sided pneumothorax.
E. Total parenteral nutrition is part of the treatment.

Q. 54
Regarding primary tumours of the lung, which of the following is false?

A. Plasma cell granuloma usually present as peripheral pulmonary mass.
B. Carcinoid tumour is a type of bronchial adenoma.
C. Bronchogenic carcinoma is rare in children.
D. Primary tumours are more common than metastatic disease.
E. Rhabdomyosarcoma is rarely seen.

Q. 55
Tumour/tumours frequently considered for metastasectomy is/are:

A. Osteogenic sarcoma.
B. Soft tissue sarcoma.
C. Wilms tumour.
D. All of the above.
E. None of the above.

Q. 56
Regarding rigid bronchoscopy, all of the following are true except:

A. It is especially for the removal of foreign bodies from the airway.
B. Neck is slightly in the antenatal position.
C. Time is a limiting factor in rigid bronchoscopy.
D. Bradycardia is one of the complications.
E. Pulmonary hypertension is a relative contraindication.

Q. 57
Regarding thoracoscopy, all of the following are true except:

A. It is used for mediastinal lesion biopsy.
B. Complete excision of bronchogenic cyst is not possible.
C. Endo GIA stapler is used for lung biopsy.
D. Plurodesis is possible using pure talc.
E. Bronchopleural fistula is a known complication after talking lung biopsy.

Q. 58
Regarding bronchogenic cysts, which of the following is false?

A. Lined by cuboidal, columnar or ciliated epithelium.
B. If communicated with airway, may produce air fluid level.
C. May develop into adenocarcinoma.
D. It is a malformation of lung, receives blood supply from one or more anomalous systemic arteries.
E. Option of treatment is enucleation, segmentectomy and lobectomy, depending upon the site.

Q. 59
Regarding pulmonary sequestration, all of the following are false except:

A. They have no bronchial communication.
B. Intralober is more common in apical segment.
C. More common on the right side.
D. Extralobers are multiple in 10 percent of cases.
E. Intralobers are less common.

Q. 60
Regarding communicating pulmonary sequestration, all the following are correct except:

A. Communication with oesophagus or stomach is well known.
B. Communication with middle oesophagus is commonest.
C. Group 1 is associated with oesophageal atresia with distal tracheoesophageal fistula.
D. X-rays show features of consolidation.

E. Anomalous arterial blood supply may be detected by Doppler ultrasound.

Q. 61
Regarding the development of lesions in mediastinum, which of the following is true?

A. Cystic hygroma from any part of mediastinum.
B. Neuroblastoma from middle mediastinum.
C. Ganglioblastoma from anterior mediastinum.
D. Teratoma from posterior mediastinum.
E. Thymoma from middle mediastinum.

Q. 62
In congenital lobar emphysema, X-ray findings may include all except:

A. There is a hyperlucent over-expanded area of lung.
B. Adjacent lung segment may be compressed or atelectasis.
C. Mediastinum is shifted on the same side.
D. Emphysematous segment may be herniated to contralateral chest.
E. There is a depression of the affected side of the diaphragm.

Q. 63
Xenon ventilation perfusion lung scan, in congenital lobar emphysema, shows which one of the following:

A. Delayed uptake and delayed washout of isotope.
B. Early uptake and delayed washout of isotopes.
C. Delayed uptake and early washout of isotopes.

D. Early uptake and early washout of isotopes.
E. Excessive blood flow from emphysematous segment.

Q. 64
Regarding cystic adenomatoid formation, all of the following are true except:

A. It is lined by psdeudocolumner epithelium.
B. There are numerous small cysts, few large cysts or bulky firm mass.
C. When it compress the oesophagus in the foetus, it develops oligohydramnios.
D. When a large mass-producing hydrop foetalis, it requires intervention in utero.
E. Newborn with respiratory distress requires high-frequency oscillatory ventilation.

Q. 65
The first phase of empyema, according to the American Thoracic Society, is:

A. Transudate.
B. Exudate.
C. Fibrinopurulent.
D. Organising.
E. None of the above.

Q. 66
Male-to-female ratio in extra-lobar sequestration is:

A. 1:1
B. 2:1
C. 3:1

D. 4:1
E. 5:1

Q. 67
Approximately what percentage of pulmonary sequestration is connected with the gastrointestinal tract?

A. 2 percent.
B. 5 percent.
C. 10 percent.
D. 20 percent.
E. 30 percent.

Q. 68
With regards to congenital lobar emphysema, all of the following are true except:

A. Tension pneumothorax is difficult to differentiate.
B. Bronchoscopy is recommended to rule out bronchial lesion.
C. It rarely involves the upper lobe.
D. There is no deficit in lung volume after operation.
E. It is attributed to dysplasia of cartilage of the affected bronchus.

Q. 69
Criteria for cystic adenomatoid malformation (CCAM) type III is:

A. Multiple larger cysts greater than 5 cm.
B. Multiple larger cysts greater than 3 cm.
C. Multiple larger cysts greater than 2 cm.

D. Multiple cysts smaller than 2 cm.
E. Multiple cysts smaller than 0.5 cm.

Q. 70
Characteristic features of extra-lobar sequestration include all of the following, except:

A. Separate from lung.
B. Mostly left side.
C. Age less than one year.
D. Mostly seen in male.
E. Venous drainage usually to pulmonary vein.

Q. 71
Regarding aspiration of chylothorax, chyle shows all of the following features, except:

A. High triglycerides.
B. Low white-cell count.
C. Significant proteins.
D. High low-density lipoproteins.
E. Cloudy in colour.

Chest Wall

Q. 72
Regarding child breast, which of the following statements is not correct?

A. Polythelia is an accessory breast.
B. Amastia is an absence of breast.
C. Mastitis neomatorum is an infectious condition.

D. Premature thelarche is breast enlargement in girls under 8 years of age.
E. Macromastia refers to large but histologically normal breast.

Q. 73
Regarding pectus excavatum, all of the following are correct except:

A. It is protrusion deformity of chest.
B. Aetiology is unknown.
C. Severity is assessed by anteroposterior diameter of chest.
D. Pulmonary function is evaluated by radio nucleotide scan.
E. It is associated with scoliosis.

Q. 74
The following are all features of Poland syndrome except:

A. Syndactyly
B. Absence of ribs
C. Athelia or amastia
D. Absence of axillary hairs
E. Absence of latissimus dorsi muscle

Q. 75
Regarding pectus excavatum, which one of the following statements is false?

A. Male-to-female ratio is 3:1.
B. Among musculoskeletal deformities, scoliosis is the most common.

C. Marfan syndrome is commonly seen.
D. Diagnosis is made in the first year of life in the majority of cases.
E. The vast majority of patients do not have symptoms.

SECTION 7

HEAD AND NECK AND SOFT TISSUE LESIONS

Head and Neck

Q. 1
Features of second branchial cyst include all except:

A. Painless.
B. Gradually increases in size.
C. Presents in upper part of posterior triangle of neck.
D. Usually presents at three to six years of age.
E. Rarely presents with stridor, sore throat and dysphagia

Q. 2
Regarding cleft lip and cleft palate, which of the following is false?

A. These constitute 80 percent of all cleft types.
B. Incidence of cleft lip is more than cleft palate.

C. Left-sided cleft lip is more common than right-sided.
D. Aetiology of clefts is multifactorial.
E. All of the above are false.

Q. 3
Regarding cleft palate, which of the following statements is true?

A. Development of primary palate related to structures posterior to incisive foramen.
B. Palatal process develops bilaterally during tenth to twelfth week of gestation.
C. Frequency in general population is 0.2 percent.
D. Repair is done during 3–4 months of age.
E. Delayed repair is indicated in Pierre Robin sequence.

Q. 4
Complications of cleft palate include all except:

A. Otitis media.
B. Respiratory tract infection.
C. Meningitis.
D. Turbinate atrophy.
E. Brain abscess.

Q. 5
Regarding Millard's procedure of cleft palate repair, which of the following is not true?

A. Rotation of medial segment.
B. Advancement of lateral segment.
C. It is flexible technique which can be modified during course of operation.

D. The cupid bow is not preserved.
E. Scar lies in good position which greatly facilitate secondary correction.

Q. 6
Regarding salivary gland, which of the following statements is false?

A. In solilithiasis, parotid gland is involved in 90 percent of cases.
B. Majority of submandibular glands are radio-opaque.
C. Ninety per cent of parotid gland stones are radiolucent.
D. Pleomorphic adenoma does not account for more than 50 percent of parotid tumours.
E. Most parotid haemangiomas regresses within two years.

Q. 7
Regarding craniofacial anomalies, all of the following are true except:

A. In craniofacial macrosomia, parotid gland is hypoplastic or absent.
B. Cranial cleft is characterised by orbital hypotelorism.
C. Treacher Collins syndrome is mandibulofacial dysostosis.
D. In Treacher Collins syndrome, there is bilateral symmetrical involvement.
E. Zygomatic bone is absent in Treacher Collins syndrome.

Q. 8
Which statement is false regarding nonsyndromic craniocynostosis?

A. Scaphocephaly develops by premature closure of multiple sutures.
B. Plagiocephaly develops by premature closure of unilateral coronal suture.
C. Brachiocephaly develops by premature closure of bilateral coronal sutures.
D. Trigonocephaly develops by premature closure of metopic sutures.
E. After linear strip craniotomy, incidence of refusion is high.

Q. 9
Regarding syndromic craniocynostosis, which of the following is false?

A. Crouzon syndrome is autosomal dominant.
B. Excorbism is a feature of Crouzon syndrome.
C. Apert's syndrome has some features like those of Crouzon syndrome.
D. In Crouzon syndrome, mental retardation is significant.
E. Symmetrical syndactyly is noted in Apert's syndrome.

Q. 10
Regarding tracheostomy, which is not true?

A. Severe epiglottitis is an indication of tracheostomy.
B. Position during tracheostomy, the neck is hyperextended.
C. Vertical incision is made over trachea at first and second tracheal ring.

D. It is essential to leave a gap around the tube to avoid post-operative surgical emphysema.
E. Persistent tracheal fistula after prolonged tracheostomy is a known complication.

Q. 11
Causes of torticollis includes all of the following, except:

A. Sternocleidomastoid tumour.
B. Cervical hemivertebrae.
C. Retropharyngeal abscess.
D. Pyloric stenosis.
E. Sandifer syndrome.

Q. 12
Regarding pathophysiology of sternocleidomastoid tumour/torticollis, all of the following are true except:

A. Breach deliveries are seen in 20–30 percent of cases.
B. It resolves spontaneously in the vast majority of cases.
C. Plagiocephally is a known complication, seen by gravity effect.
D. Bilateral facial hypoplasia has been seen.
E. Fibrous replacement of muscle bundle has seen.

Q. 13
Regarding operative treatment of sternocleidomastoid tumour/torticollis, all of the following are true except:

A. Indication of surgery is sternocleidomastoid tightening, limiting head rotation beyond 3 months of age.
B. Incision is given 1 cm above the sternal and clavicular head of sternocleidomastoid muscle.

C. Full range of movement normally achieved within one week of surgery.
D. Recurrent torticollis is a known complication.
E. Patient should be followed after surgery until torticollis has been resolved completely.

Q. 14
The most common brachial anomalies are:

A. First branchial anomalies.
B. Second branchial anomalies.
C. Third branchial anomalies.
D. Fourth branchial anomalies.
E. Fifth branchial anomalies.

Q. 15
Regarding thyroglossal duct cyst, which one is false?

A. Most common congenital midline neck mass.
B. Enlarged lymph node is one of the differential diagnoses.
C. Excision is accompanied with excision of central part of hyoid bone.
D. One percent develop carcinoma, mostly papillary.
E. It is derivative of second branchial arch.

Q. 16
With regards to solitary thyroid nodule, all are false except:

A. It is common in children as compared to adults.
B. When present they are more likely to be benign.
C. Most are well differentiated papillary carcinoma.

D. Cancers occur most frequently between 5 and 10 years of age.
E. Boys are affected more than girls.

Soft Tissue Lesions

Q. 17
Regarding congenital giant hairy Nevus most perfect answer among following is:

A. It is malpositioning of otherwise normal structure.
B. It is regional absence of normal tissue.
C. It is an aberration of tissue composition.
D. All of the above are correct.
E. None of the above is correct.

Q. 18
Regarding syndactyly, which of the following is true?

A. It is a transverse arrest of development.
B. It is a longitudinal deficiency.
C. It is a failure of differentiation.
D. It is commonly seen between the index and middle finger.
E. Syndromic features of syndactyly include Down syndrome.

Q. 19
Regarding deformities of digits, which of the following is false?

A. Clinodactyly means medial or lateral curve of the digit.
B. In polydactyly, central digit duplication is the most common.

C. Mirror hand possess seven or eight digits.
D. Macrodactyly is associated with neurofibromatosis.
E. Brachydactyly means shortened digits.

Q. 20
The cause of conjoint twin is:

A. Zygote divided in the first to seventh day of gestation.
B. Two separate ova are fertilised.
C. Inner cell mass incompletely divides.
D. All of the above.
E. None of the above.

Q. 21
The commonest type of conjoint twin is

A. Thoracopagus.
B. Omphalopagus.
C. Pyopagus.
D. Ischiopagus.
E. Craniopagus.

Q. 22
Regarding organs potentially involved in Ischiopagus, which of the following groups is most perfect.

A. Heart, liver and intestine.
B. Liver, biliary tract and intestine.
C. Spine, rectum and genitourinary tract.
D. Pelvis, intestine, genitourinary tract and liver.
E. Brain.

SECTION 8

ORTHOPEDIC

Digital Malformation

Q. 1
Regarding digital malformation, all of the following are false except:

   A. Syndactyly develops by programmed cell death in between digits.
   B. In symbrachydactyly, digits are short.
   C. In achrocephlodactyly, there is complete syndactyly of all four limbs.
   D. Syndactyly is also seen in Poland syndrome.
   E. Superdigit is a form of syndactyly.

Q. 2
Regarding syndactyly, all of the following are true except:

   A. Syndactyly of hand is usually separated unless there is definitive contraindication.

B. First web space should always be separated to provide independent functioning thumb.
C. Two years is a good age if child is fit.
D. Simple syndactyly of smaller toe is of no functional importance and should not be divided in childhood.
E. Zigzag scar causes less contracture than longitudinal scar on volar aspect of fingers.

Spina Bifida

Q. 3
Regarding spina bifida, all of the following are false except:

A. In spinabifida occulta, neural deficit may or may not be at birth; it may develop at any age but often before one year of age.
B. Spina bifida aperta has no apparent lesion on back but there is bifid spine.
C. Meningomylocele represents a failure of fusion of neural folds.
D. Lipomeningocele fat is not extended in spinal canal.
E. Meningocele contains spinal elements.

Q. 4
Meningocele may be associated with all of the following except:

A. Chiari II malformation.
B. Microcephaly.
C. Genitourinary abnormality.
D. Abnormality of lips.
E. Abnormality of foot.

Q. 5
Which is false about Chiari II malformation.

A. It may be symptomatic in the first few months of life.
B. There is downward displacement of vermis in the cervical spinal cord.
C. There is compression of brain stem and spinal cord.
D. Features are apnea, stridor and high-pitched cry.
E. Upper crania nerve paresis.

Telipes Equinovarus

Q. 6
The features of clubfoot (telipes equinovarus) include all except:

A. Planter flexion.
B. Lateral deviation (Concave lateral border of foot).
C. Short foot.
D. Tightening of Achilles tendon.
E. Small heal.

Q. 7
Extrinsic causes of telipes equinovarus include all except:

A. Firstborn child.
B. Large infant with small mother.
C. Amniotic constricting band.
D. Oligohydramnios.
E. Meningomylocele.

Q. 8
Regarding pathology of talipes equinovarus, which of the following is false?

A. It is well understood.
B. Talus is longer than normal.
C. Talonavicular joint is medially deviated.
D. Achilles tendon is contracted.
E. Posterior tibial tendon is contracted.

Q. 9
Regarding treatment of talipes equinovarus, which one is false?

A. Treatment begins soon after birth.
B. First, correct the medial deviation of talonavicular joint.
C. Surgery, if required, should be done in preschool age.
D. In mildest residual deformity, posterior release is required only.
E. Posterior tibial artery and nerve is isolated during surgery (in posteromedial release).

Q. 10
The following are complications of surgical correction of talipes equinovarus except:

A. Injury to posterior tibial nerve.
B. Injury to common peroneal nerve.
C. Injury to sural nerve.
D. Injury to posterior tibial artery.
E. Contracture.

Developmental Dysplasia of Hip

Q. 11
The possible causes of developmental dysplasia (DDH) of hip include all except:

A. Ligamentous stiffness.
B. Abnormal intrauterine position.
C. Foetal crowding.
D. Breech position.
E. Oligohydramnios.

Q. 12
Regarding Barlow and Ortoloni test for DDH, all of the following are correct except:

A. It is useful up to three months of age.
B. Barlow is for hip instability and Ortoloni is for dislocation.
C. In Barlow, adduct the hip and apply downward pressure on knee.
D. Clunking sensation is felt during Barlow manoeuvre.
E. Ortoloni test shows a hip that is dislocated but reducible.

Q. 13
In walking child, the developmental dysplasia of hip (DDH) shows all of the following except:

A. Excessive kyphosis.
B. Pelvic obliquity.
C. Unequal length.
D. Contracture of hip flexors.
E. Insufficient abductors.

Q. 14
Regarding diagnosis of developmental dysplasia of hip (DDH), all of the following are correct, except:

A. Physical examination (Barlow and Ortoloni) test for diagnosis is used up to 6 months of age.
B. Ultrasound is useful up to 6 months of age.
C. X-rays are useful up to 6 months of age.
D. Wedding gait is seen in bilateral hip dislocation.
E. Contrast orthography is gold slandered but it is invasive and needs investigation.

Q. 15
Regarding pathoanotomy of developmental dysplasia of hip, which one is false?

A. Contracture of iliopsoas.
B. Atrophy of acetabulum.
C. Thickening of transverse acetabular ligament.
D. Elongation of ligamentous teres.
E. Proliferation of fibro fatty tissue, filling of depth of acetabulum.

Q. 16
Regarding management of developmental dysplasia of hip, all of the following are correct, except:

A. It is useful in older children.
B. Goal is to remove obstacle that prevents seating of femoral head in acetabulum and to make hip stable.
C. Medial approach is most commonly used.
D. Femoral osteotomy may be required.
E. Pelvis osteotomy may be required.

Septic Arthritis

Q. 17
Regarding septic arthritis, all of the following are correct except:

A. Pseudo paralysis of limb.
B. String sign of joint fluid indicates that the normal viscosity is lost.
C. Can results in permanent loss of joint if ignored beyond 24 hours.
D. H-influenza is the commonest organism involved in septic arthritis.
E. Gonococci is involved in neonate septic arthritis.

Osteomylitis

Q. 18
Regarding osteomyelitis, all the following are false except:

A. Group B-streptococcus is the commonest organism involved.
B. Pseudomonas is specifically involved in osteomyelitis in sickle cell patients.
C. When infection is locally confined but is not eradicated, it results in Brodie's abscess.
D. Necrotic bone is called involucrum.
E. New bone formed around dead bone is called sequestrum.

Q. 19
In osteomyelitis, all of the following are true except:

A. The commonest bones involved are femur and tibia.
B. On X-rays, initially there are no bony changes.
C. The first change on X-rays is increase in bone density.
D. Ultrasound may also useful in identifying and localising subperiosteal abscess.
E. Bone infarction appears as cold spot rather than hot on bone scan.

Femur Fracture

Q. 20
Disadvantages of early spica cast for femur fracture include all except:

A. Shortening.
B. Problem of transposition.
C. Cast soakage and breakage.
D. Cleaning difficulties.
E. Prolonged hospital stay.

Q. 21
Disadvantages of skeletal traction in femoral fracture include all except:

A. Risk of infection.
B. Need for anaesthesia.
C. Traction possible only for short period.
D. Risk of physical injury.
E. Long hospital stay.

Q. 22
Disadvantages of external fixator for femoral fracture includes all of the following, except:

- A. Pin tract infection.
- B. Difficult wound care in compound fracture.
- C. Refracture after removal.
- D. Angular and rotational deformity.
- E. Heterotrophic ossification around pin tract.

Q. 23
Internal fixation in fracture femur has the following advantages, except:

- A. Stable reduction.
- B. Less chances of infection.
- C. Early mobilisation.
- D. Short hospital stay.
- E. Cost effectiveness.

Q. 24
Early complications of fracture femur include all except:

- A. Pseudoarthrosis.
- B. Soft tissue injury.
- C. Vascular injury
- D. Fat embolism.
- E. Crush limb syndrome.

Q. 25
The following are late complications of femur fracture except:

A. Compartment syndrome.
B. malunion.
C. Non-union.
D. Knee stiffness.
E. Volkmann ischemic contracture.

Ingrown Toenail

Q. 26
Regarding aetiology ingrown toenail, which of the following statements is false?

A. Ill-fitting footwear.
B. Bad nail care.
C. Tight stalking and hyperhidrosis.
D. Diabetics and immunosuppressive.
E. None of the above.

Q. 27
Regarding grading of ingrown toenails, which statement is false?

A. Grade I: pain and redness and slight swelling of nail.
B. Grade II: features of grade I accompanied by infection suppuration.
C. Grade III: features grade I and II with formation of granulation tissue.
D. None of the above.
E. All of the above.

Q. 28
Regarding management of ingrown toenails, all of the following are correct except:

A. Indicated in grade III and some grade II presentation.
B. Operation is indicated when there are physical signs of ischaemia.
C. X-rays are needed if subungual exocytosis or bony abnormality is suspected.
D. Radioisotope scan is needed if osteomyelitis is suspected.
E. MRI is needed if subungual glomus tumour is suspected.

Q. 29
Regarding wedge resection for ingrown toenails, all of the following are true except:

A. Recovery time is two weeks to two months.
B. Oral or topical antibiotics should be used for a week.
C. Special soaks should be used for a week.
D. If ingrown toenail is bilateral, bilateral wedge resection can be done.
E. Phenol ablation of nail matrix at the site of resection increases the recurrence rate.

SECTION 9

TRAUMA

Abdominal Trauma

Q. 1
Peritoneal lavage is considered positive if lavage effluent contains following except:

- A. Blood.
- B. Bacteria/faeces.
- C. Bile.
- D. Amylase.
- E. Lipase.

Q. 2
In the management of penetrating abdominal trauma (stab wound), which one is not correct.

- A. Stab wound does not need local wound exploration.
- B. Indication of laparotomy includes unstable patient, unexplained blood loss and signs of peritonitis.

C. Positive peritoneal lavage needs laparotomy.
D. Negative peritoneal lavage with signs of peritonitis needs laparotomy.
E. If intact posterior fascia, patient can be discharged.

Q. 3
After four blood transfusions, the following should all be administered except:

A. Fresh frozen plasma.
B. Platelets.
C. Magnesium.
D. Calcium.
E. Sodium bicarbonate.

Q. 4
In the management of diaphragmatic injury due to blunt abdominal trauma, which of the following is false?

A. Transthoracic approach is preferable in acute cases.
B. Two layered closure is preferable.
C. Non-absorbable suture is preferable.
D. In stable patient GIT series and ultrasound is helpful.
E. X-rays show shifting of mediastinum to opposite side.

Q. 5
Regarding gastric perforation in trauma, all are correct except:

A. It is more common in children than in adults.
B. Peritoneal lavage is indicated in comatose patient.
C. Rupture usually occurs in on the greater curvature.
D. Defect is best closed in two layers.

E. Percutaneous gastrostomy is considered if extensive contamination has occurred or other injury is present.

Q. 6
In traumatic intestinal perforation, all of the following are false except:

A. Mobile portion of intestine is more prone to perforation.
B. Perforation mostly occurs on mesenteric border.
C. CT scan is non-diagnostic.
D. Best repair is by simple closure.
E. Physiological stability may necessitate exteriorization.

Q. 7
Regarding splenic trauma, which of the following is false?

A. Unique radial segmental blood supply permits resection and repair of both large and small portion of spleen.
B. Pain radiograph shows medial gastric displacement.
C. Decision of laparotomy based on extent of injury as shown on CT.
D. There are many techniques of splenoraphy.
E. During laparotomy, unreasonable prolongation of surgery in patient with multiple trauma is one of the indications of splenectomy.

Q. 8
Regarding post splenectomy treatment, all of the following are correct except:

A. Vaccination against H-Influenza.
B. Vaccination against meningococcus.

C. Vaccination against streptococcus.
D. Prophylactic antibiotic with penicillin.
E. Medical Alert tag.

Q. 9
Regarding pancreatic and duodenal injury, all of the following are false except:

A. Pancreas and duodenum are retroperitoneal, so fully protected.
B. Blunt trauma is more common cause than penetrating trauma.
C. X-rays show air around left kidney.
D. Serum amylase and lipase levels are low.
E. Positive peritoneal lavage for bile and amylase is specific for pancreaticoduodenal injury.

Q. 10
Regarding pseudopancreatic cyst, which of the following is true?

A. It is not a consequence of inflammatory process.
B. It is not a consequence of direct trauma to duct system.
C. Manifests within 3–4 weeks of injury.
D. Treatment is medical within first week.
E. Mostly resolves spontaneously and does not require drainage.

Q. 11
Regarding hepatic trauma, which of the following is not true?

A. Penetrating trauma is less common than blunt.
B. CT scan helps in diagnosis.

C. Non-operative treatment depends upon physiological stability.
D. Non-expending haematoma resolve spontaneously.
E. All above statements are false.

Q. 12
Management of diffuse parenchymal bleeding in hepatic trauma include all except:

A. Cauterization.
B. Manual pressure.
C. Direct ligation of vessel.
D. Placement of radivac drain.
E. General management of patient for haemodynamic stability.

Q. 13
Management of complication, after acute management of liver injury, all are true except:

A. Monthly observation for stable haematoma.
B. Roux-en-Y hepaticojejunostomy for bile duct strictures.
C. External drainage of haemobilia (bleeding in biliary tree), if arteriogram shows aneurysm.
D. External drainage of hepatic abscess.
E. Cholecystectomy for gallbladder injury.

Q. 14
Grade IV hepatic injury is labelled with which of the following features?

A. Laceration 1 cm deep.
B. Bi-lobar tissue maceration and devascularisation.

C. Laceration 3–10 cm deep.
D. Laceration more than 10 cm deep.
E. Laceration 1–3 cm deep.

Q. 15
Regarding classification of pancreatic injury, which of the following statements is false?

A. Class I injury is contusion and laceration without ductal injury.
B. Class II injury is distal transection or parenchymal injury with probable ductal injury.
C. Proximal transection or parenchymal injury with probable ductal injury.
D. Combined pancreatic and duodenal injury.
E. All of the above are false statements.

Urogenital Injury

Q. 16
Regarding urethral injury all of the following are false except:

A. Posterior urethral injury is most commonly caused by penetrating trauma.
B. Straddle injury causes anterior urethral trauma.
C. Blood at urethral meatus is less common finding.
D. Urethral contusion is considered as grade II urethral injury.
E. Partial disruption is considered as grade II urethral injury.

Q. 17
Regarding management of urethral injuries, which one is true?

A. Pass folly's catheter in complex anterior urethral injuries.
B. Delayed primary realignment causes more bleeding.
C. Delayed primary realignment is contraindicated in boys with disruption of bladder neck.
D. Secondary reconstruction is done after one month.
E. Secondary reconstruction has more incidence of impotency and incontinence.

Q. 18
Regarding long-term sequelae of urethral injury, all of the following are false except:

A. Impotence is more common than urethral stricture.
B. Urinary incontinence is more common than impotence.
C. Bladder neck mechanism is not important to avoid retrograde ejaculation.
D. Impotence is caused by injury to nerve to erigentes.
E. Urethral stricture is not the direct consequence of trauma.

Q. 19
On the organ-injury-severity scale for the kidney, which grade would you label a laceration more than one centimetre parenchymal deep in the renal cortex without collecting system rupture or urinary extravasation?

A. Grade I.
B. Grade II.
C. Grade III.

D. Grade IV.
E. Grade V.

Q. 20
In which of the following situation can we diagnose grade IV ureteral injury.

A. Avulsion with more than 2 cm devascularisation.
B. Contusion or haematoma.
C. Less than 50 percent transection.
D. More than 50per cent transection.
E. All of the above are false.

Q. 21
You can label grade IV urethral injury in case of the following feature.

A. Complete transection with more than 2 cm urethral separation.
B. Partial disruption.
C. Contusion.
D. Complete disruption with less than 2 cm urethral separation.
E. Stretch injury.

Burn

Q. 22
In the management of burns, all of the following are false except:

A. Fifty per cent have about a fifty per cent survival rate.
B. Parkland formula is 2 ml/kg/ percent of burned surface are.

C. Fifty per cent of Parkland formula is given in the first 6 hours.
D. In a one-year-old child, head constitutes 19 percent.
E. In a four-year-old child, one lower limb constitutes 18 percent.

Q. 23
In relation to topical antimicrobials used in burns, all are false except:

A. Silver sulphadiazine is a painful application.
B. Mefenide acetate does not penetrate eschar.
C. Silver nitrate penetrates eschar.
D. Povidone iodine is a painful application.
E. Gentamicin is narrow spectrum.

Q. 24
Regarding management of infection in burn, all are true except:

A. Purpose of topical antibiotic is to keep bacteria below 100 organism/gram of tissue.
B. If the level of bacteria is 105/gram of tissue, a change in the antibiotic is warranted.
C. Bacteria invasion is suspected when bacterial count is 1015/gram of tissue.
D. Hypothermia is a feature of septicaemia.
E. In burn patients, infection may be in wound, lung and urine or at cannula site.

Q. 25
In burn patient, which of the following is false?

A. In 40 percent of total burn surface area (TBSA), there is a 50–100 percent increase in BMR (basal metabolic rate).
B. Increase in catecholamine is cause of necrotising enterocolitis.
C. Prolonged growth arrest noted in first year.
D. A decrease in growth hormones and IGF-I strongly suggests that administration of human growth hormones would be advantageous.
E. All of the above are false.

Q. 26
Characteristics of full-thickness skin burn include all except:

A. All viable epithelium are destroyed.
B. Wound is often pink with bullae.
C. There is thrombosed superficial vein.
D. There is no sensation.
E. It requires skin grafting.

Q. 27
Acid burn causes all of the following except:

A. Saponification of fat.
B. Electrolyte abnormalities.
C. Renal failure.
D. Intravascular haemolysis
E. RDS (respiratory distress)

Q. 28
Regarding high-voltage electric current, all of the following are true except:

A. Deep-tissue destruction is produced by heat generated by electric resistance of tissues.
B. Bone injury is common.
C. If facial compartmental pressure is increased, do eschorotomy to prevent limb.
D. Haemochromogen is present in urine.
E. Delayed complication includes neurological disorder, cataracts and paralysis.

Q. 29
Regarding inhalation injury in burn patient, all of the following are true except:

A. Increase in vasoactive amines causes pulmonary oedema.
B. We label carbon monoxide poisoning if carboxy haemoglobin increases to 3 percent.
C. Twenty per cent acetyl cysteine nebuliser solution is used.
D. Nebulise with heparin (5000–10,000 U) with 3 ml of normal saline every 4 hours.
E. High flow of humidified oxygen is required.

Q. 30
Inhalation injury in burn has mortality of approximately.

A. 20 percent.
B. 30 percent.
C. 40 percent.

D. 50 percent.
E. 60 percent.

Thoracic Trauma

Q. 31
Regarding thoracic injury, the following are immediate life-threatening injuries except:

    A. Pulmonary contusion.
    B. Airway obstruction.
    C. Tension pneumothorax.
    D. Massive haemothorax.
    E. Cardiac tamponade.

Q. 32
Which one is the commonest thoracic injury?

    A. Pneumothorax.
    B. Lung contusion.
    C. Haemothorax.
    D. Rib fracture.
    E. Ruptured diaphragm.

Q. 33
All of the following are indication for emergency thoracotomy except:

    A. Penetrating wound of heart and great vessels.
    B. Massive or continuous intrathoracic bleed.
    C. Tension pneumothorax.
    D. Aortogram showing aorta or major branch injury.
    E. Cardiac tamponade.

Q. 34
Regarding chest injury, which of the following signs is *not* correlated with the condition?

   A. Noisy breathing results from foreign material blood, vomitus or mucus in the airway.
   B. Tracheal deviation implies massive haemothorax.
   C. Hoarseness indicates tension pneumothorax.
   D. Surgical emphysema suggests tracheal or bronchial laceration or oesophageal perforation.
   E. Increased JVP, decreased blood pressure and increased pulses paradoxes ≥10 mm Hg, implies cardiac tamponade.

Q. 35
The following is ECMO exclusion criteria except:

   A. Grade II intraventricular haemorrhage.
   B. Weight less than 2 kg.
   C. Severe chromosomal abnormalities.
   D. Reversible cardiovascular failure.
   E. Cyanotic heart disease.

Child Abuse

Q. 36
Regarding child abuse, which of the following is false?

   A. Fractures at various stages of healing is seen in shaken baby syndrome.
   B. Abdominal injury is uncommon in abused child.
   C. Long bone fracture is more common than skull fracture.

D. Burn in abused children, most victims are less than two years.
E. In the absence of major trauma or pre-existing disease, rib fractures in infants must be considered as evidence of no accidental injury.

Birth Trauma

Q. 37
Which one is false about birth injuries?

A. In Erb's palsy, there is lack of shoulder motion.
B. In Klumpke's palsy, there is lack of wrist movement.
C. Horner's syndrome is associated with Klumpke's paralysis.
D. Phrenic nerve injury is associated with Erb's palsy.
E. Among fracture, humerus fracture is most common in birth injuries.

SECTION 10

ONCOLOGY

General Oncology

Q. 1
Regarding paediatric oncology, all of the following are true except:

A. Lymphoma is commonest malignancy.
B. Viral oncogene is pathogen.
C. Carcinogenesis occurs either through activation of growth-promoting oncogene or the loss of growth regulating tumour suppressor gene.
D. Diploid chromosomes show good prognosis, while hyperlipoid chromosomes show bad prognosis.
E. Cancer can result from genetic effects that alter a single cell.

Q. 2
All of the following are principles of radiation therapy, except:

A. Radiosensitivity of the tumour cells should be more than the surrounding normal cells.
B. The higher the energy, the deeper the ionizing radiation penetration.
C. The lesser the mitotic activity, the more the sensitivity to radiation.
D. Oxygenated tissues are much more sensitive to radiation than hypoxic tissues.
E. Minimise the exposure of normal tissues to radiation.

Q. 3
Regarding side effects of chemotherapeutic drugs, all of the following are correct except:

A. Cisplatin is nephrotoxic.
B. Methotrexate causes restrictive lung disease.
C. Anthramycin is cardiotoxic.
D. Dactinomycin causes GIT mucositis and diarrhoea.
E. Bone marrow is affected by most of chemotherapeutic drugs.

Central Nervous System Tumour

Q. 4
The commonest central nervous tumour is:

A. Astrocytoma.
B. Craniophrangioma.
C. Meningioma.

D. Primitive neuroectodermal tumour (PNET).
E. Ependimoma.

Q. 5
The commonest site of distribution of brain tumour is:

A. Supratentorial hemispheric.
B. Infratentorial.
C. Supratentorial.
D. Suprasellar.
E. Pineal region.

Q. 6
Regarding diagnostic study of CNS tumour, all of the following are correct except:

A. CT scan is better than MRI.
B. Intramural calcification in teratoma is seen poorly on MRI.
C. CSF can shows high alpha-fetoprotein and beta-HCG in germ cell tumour.
D. Embolization is required preoperatively.
E. Post-operative imaging is required to assess the extent of tumour resection and complication like haematoma and hydrocephalus.

Q. 7
Regarding central nervous tumour all of the following are correct except:

A. Astrocytoma is usually malignant.
B. Ependimoma is usually benign.

C. Diffuse intrinsic pontine glioma is not amenable to surgical resection.
D. Atypical teratoma is highly malignant.
E. Craniopharyngioma is excised through trans-sphenoid approach.

Q. 8
Regarding vascular malformation of brain, which of the following is false?

A. For aneurysm, surgery is usually always needed.
B. Cavernous haemangioma if symptomatic requires surgery.
C. Incidental venous angioma should not be treated.
D. For large arteriovenous malformation, preoperative embolization is required.
E. Clipping of feeding vessels is ideal treatment for arteriovenous malformation.

Q. 9
Regarding principles of chemotherapy, all of the following are false except:

A. Single-agent chemotherapy is better than combined chemotherapy.
B. Recovery of normal tissue takes average 7 days after chemotherapy, so interval is required.
C. Dose of chemotherapy is administered as minimum as possible.

D. Continuous administration for longer duration of chemotherapy is better than shorter the duration of administration.
E. Neoadjuvant chemotherapy is administered for residual disease after excision of tumour.

Teratoma and Germ Cell Tumour

Q. 10
Regarding germ cell tumour all of the following are correct except:

A. Germ cells develop from pluripotent cells.
B. Dysgerminoma is a hormone secretion tumour.
C. Immature teratoma is a premature condition.
D. Yolk sac endodermal sinus tumour develops from intraembryonic differentiation.
E. Trophoblastic choriocarcinoma is a hormone-secreting tumour.

Q. 11
Which of the following statements regarding type of sacrococcygeal teratoma is false?

A. Type I is predominantly external with minimum presacral component.
B. Type II is external with significant intrapelvic component.
C. Type III is external with predominant pelvic mass with extension into the abdomen.
D. Type IV is entirely presacral with external presentation.
E. All of the above are false.

Q. 12
Alpha-fetoprotein is high in all of the following conditions except:

   A. Embryonal carcinoma.
   B. Endodermal sinus tumour
   C. Seminoma.
   D. Hepatic malignancy.
   E. Hypothyroidism.

Q. 13
In all of the following conditions, Beta HCG is high except:

   A. Choriocarcinoma.
   B. Hydatidiform mole.
   C. Germ cell tumour without trophoblastic component.
   D. Hepatoma.
   E. Hepatoblastoma.

Q. 14
The commonest site of germ cell tumour is:

   A. Sacrococcygeal.
   B. Mediastinal.
   C. Abdominal.
   D. Ovarian.
   E. Testicular.

Q. 15
Factors associated with worst prognosis in malignant germ cell tumour include all except:

   A. An extragonadal location.
   B. Age less than 11 years.

C. Extent of disease.
D. Inability to perform complete resection.
E. Germinoma or mixed germ cell tumour.

Q. 16
Regarding teratoma in children, all of the following are true except:

A. Contains all the three germ layer.
B. Tumour size does not relate to the risk of malignancy.
C. Children less than two years of age risk of malignancy is 10–20 percent.
D. After 2 years of age, risk of malignancy is almost 80 percent.
E. Radiation is commonly used in this disease.

Q. 17
Which of the following is not germ cell tumour.

A. Leydig cell.
B. Yolk sac.
C. Mixed germ cell tumour.
D. Seminoma.
E. Teratoma.

Q. 18
Which of the following is commonest testicular tumour?

A. Rhabdomyosarcoma.
B. Yolk sac tumour.
C. Teratoma.
D. Mixed germ cell tumour.
E. Seminoma.

Sarcoma

Q. 19
Regarding rhabdomyosarcoma, which of the following is false?

A. It arises from embryonic mesenchyme.
B. It has the potential to differentiate into smooth muscle.
C. It accounts 15 percent of solid tumours.
D. It accounts 50 percent of soft tissue sarcoma.
E. It is sensitive to chemotherapy and radiotherapy.

Q. 20
The commonest site of rhabdomyosarcoma is:

A. Head and neck.
B. Genitourinary.
C. Prostate.
D. Limbs.
E. Chest.

Q. 21
Commonest histological type of rhabdomyosarcoma is:

A. Alveolar.
B. Botroid.
C. Embryonal.
D. Pleomorphic.
E. Undifferentiated

Q. 22
Which one of rhabdomyosarcoma has the best prognosis?

A. Alveolar.
B. Pleomorphic.
C. Embryonal.
D. Spindle cell.
E. Botroid.

Q. 23
Which of the following comes in category IIC, according to clinical group classification of rhabdomyosarcoma?

A. Microscopic residual tumour at primary site and pathological negative lymph node.
B. Non-residual tumour at primary site and pathological positive lymph node.
C. Gross residual.
D. Distant metastasis.
E. None of the above.

Q. 24
All of the following are considered unfavourable site for rhabdomyosarcoma except:

A. Parameningeal head and neck.
B. Bladder.
C. Prostate.
D. Limb.
E. Orbit.

Q. 25
Regarding sarcoma of bone in children, which of the following statements is not true?

A. Sarcoma of bone comprises 5 percent of all malignant paediatric tumours.
B. For osteosarcoma of long bones, long-term survival is less than 30 per cent.
C. Evan's sarcoma is small, blue round cell tumour.
D. Ewing's sarcoma local control rate is 90 percent.
E. Ewing's sarcoma is chemo-sensitive.

Ovarian Lesions

Q. 26
Regarding ovarian cyst and tumour, all of the following are correct except:

A. Preconscious puberty may occurs in luteal cyst.
B. Elevated oestrogen is cause of preconscious puberty.
C. High beta HCG is cause of preconscious puberty.
D. Peutz-Jegher syndrome is associated with corpus luteal cyst.
E. Gross residual is considered as stage III germ cell tumour.

Q. 27
Regarding neoplastic ovarian cyst, which of the following statements is false?

A. Among epithelial tumours, 10 per cent are malignant.
B. Sertoli-Leydig cell tumour may produce alpha-fetoprotein.

C. Fibroma are most common among sex cord stromal tumour.
D. Mucinous are epithelial variety of tumour.
E. Sclerosing stromal tumour associated with Chediak-Higashi syndrome.

Q. 28
Regarding germ cell tumour of ovary, all of the following statements are true except:

A. Mature teratoma are more common than immature teratoma.
B. Dysgerminoma is most common among malignant ovarian tumour.
C. Choriocarcinoma shows high alpha-fetoprotein.
D. Gonadoblastoma develops from dysgenetic gonads.
E. Contralateral ovary should be examined at the time of surgery.

Liver Tumours

Q. 29
Which one of the following is the most common liver tumour?

A. Hepatocellular carcinoma.
B. Hepatoblastoma.
C. Sarcoma.
D. Mesenchymal hamartoma.
E. Adenoma.

Q. 30
What is the mean age of children with hepatoblastoma?

A. 3.5 years.
B. 5.5 years.
C. 7.5 years.
D. 9.5 years.
E. 11.5 years.

Q. 31
Regarding diagnostic studies in hepatic tumours, all of the following are correct except:

A. MRI is more accurate in diagnosis than CT scan.
B. CT scan of the chest is indicated to see metastatic disease.
C. Arteriography is used in therapy for chemoembolization and intra-arterial infusion of cytotoxic drugs.
D. Alpha-fetoprotein has diagnostic value.
E. Thrombocytosis develops because of release of cytokines from tumour.

Q. 32
Regarding histological subtypes of hepatoblastoma, which of the following statements is correct?

A. Small cell is more common than foetal.
B. Macrotrabacular is more common than embryonal.
C. Teratoid is more common than non-teratoid.
D. Foetal is more common than teratoid.
E. Epithelial and mixed epithelial are not subtypes of hepatoblastoma.

Q. 33
Regarding pathology of hepatoblastoma, which of the following statements is false?

A. Usually it is bulky and solitary mass.
B. It is surrounded by pseudocapsule.
C. Bilober disease is common.
D. Aneuploid lesion has better prognosis than diploid tumour.
E. Increased mitotic activity shows poor prognosis.

Q. 34
With regard to hepatic tumour in children, which of the following is not true?

A. Primary tumour of liver is uncommon.
B. Forty per cent of primary liver tumours are malignant.
C. Hepatoblastoma is the most common primary liver tumour in children.
D. Hepatoblastoma affects boys as frequently as girls.
E. Right lobe is more commonly involved.

Wilms Tumour

Q. 35
Regarding Wilms tumour, all of the following are false except:

A. Tumour produces alpha-fetoprotein, which causes hypertension.
B. WT1 is an oncogene, which causes tumour development.
C. Beta HCG is present in urine and has prognostic value.
D. Stage I disease is limited to the capsule.
E. Bilateral renal involvement is stage IV disease.

Q. 36
What percentage of Wilms tumour are bilateral?

A. 1–5 percent.
B. 5–10 percent.
C. 10–15 percent.
D. 15–20 percent.
E. 20–25 percent.

Q. 37
What is survival rate for bilateral Wilms tumour?

A. 25 percent.
B. 50 percent.
C. 75 percent.
D. 100 percent.
E. 0 percent.

Lymphoma

Q. 38
Features of cervical lymphadenitis due to lymphoma include all except:

A. Discharging sinus.
B. Longer duration.
C. No pain.
D. Weight loss.
E. Other enlarge lymph nodes in the body.

Q. 39
Regarding undifferentiated lymphoma, which one is not correct?

A. It is variety of non-Hodgkin lymphoma.
B. It develops from B cells.
C. Burkitt's lymphoma is its one variety.
D. The majority of these present as thymic or mediastinal masses.
E. Chemotherapy is primary modality of treatment.

Q. 40
Regarding lymphoblastic lymphoma which one of the following statements is false?

A. It is a variety of non-Hodgkin lymphoma.
B. It originates from T cells.
C. Non-Burkitt lymphoma is one of the varieties.
D. The majority of these present as thymic or mediastinal masses.
E. Chemotherapy is the primary modality of treatment.

Q. 41
Which of the following develops from posterior mediastinum?

A. Thymoma.
B. Lymphoma.
C. Neuroblastoma.
D. Teratoma.
E. Dermoid cyst.

Q. 42
Which one is the commonest mediastinal mass?

A. Neurogenic tumour, such as neuroblastoma and others.
B. Lymphoma.
C. Germ cell tumour.
D. Mesenchymal tumour.
E. Thymic lesion.

Q. 43
Regarding diagnosis and management of mediastinal masses, which of the following statements is not true?

A. CT is superior with ability to define to define calcification within the mass.
B. Oesophagogram is indicated in foregut duplication.
C. Urinary catecholamine for anterior mediastinal masses.
D. Pre-operative alpha fetoprotein and beta HCG particularly for anterior mediastinal masses.
E. Common approach for anterior mediastinal masses is median sternotomy.

Q. 44
With regard to lymphoma, what is false?

A. It is a variety of small blue cell tumour.
B. C-myc proto-oncogene translocation between chromosomes number 14 and 18 is associated with Burkitt's lymphoma.
C. Almost all intestinal lymphoma are non-Hodgkin's type.
D. Lymphoblastic lymphoma occurs in predominantly in anterior mediastinum.

E. It is associated with increases serum alpha-fetoprotein.

Q. 45
Small round cell tumours include all except:

A. Lymphoma.
B. Primary neuroectodermal tumour.
C. Rhabdomyosarcoma.
D. Hepatoblastoma.
E. Ewing's sarcoma.

Pheochromocytoma

Q. 46
Which one is the most common site among following for extra-adrenal pheochromocytoma?

A. Lymph node.
B. Liver.
C. Lung.
D. Bone.
E. Organ of Zuckerkandl.

Q. 47
In comparison of adult pheochromocytoma, paediatric pheochromocytoma has all of the following features except:

A. More malignant.
B. More bilaterally.
C. More sustained hypertension.
D. More familial pattern.
E. More extra-adrenal site.

Q. 48
Pheochromocytoma shows following clinical feature except:

A. Headache.
B. Polyuria.
C. Polydipsia.
D. Hypotension.
E. Hyperglycaemia.

Q. 49
With regards to pheochromocytoma in children, all are true except:

A. It is commonly bilateral.
B. The tumour rarely involves blood vessels.
C. The hypertension is typically sustained rather than episodic.
D. Thirty per cent are malignant.
E. Thirty per cent have extra-adrenal disease.

Q. 50
Scan for diagnosis of pheochromocytoma is

A. DTPS.
B. DMSA.
C. MAG 3.
D. HIDA.
E. MIBG.

Neuroblastoma

Q. 51
Regarding features of neuroblastoma, all of the following are false except:

A. Proptosis because of bleeding in eyeball.
B. Hypertension because of cortisol secretion.
C. Diarrhoea because of VIP (vasoactive intestinal polypeptide) secretion.
D. Bleeding because of thrombocytosis.
E. Horner's syndrome, when it arises from the adrenal gland.

Q. 52
All of the following are bad prognostic factors of neuroblastoma except:

A. Age more than one year.
B. Stage IV-S.
C. When adrenal gland is the site of development.
D. Elevated serum ferritin level.
E. Stoma poor Shimada histology.

Q. 53
Which of the following mediastinal mass shows features of Horner's syndrome.

A. Lymphoma.
B. Teratoma.
C. Thymic hyperplasia.
D. Neuroblastoma.
E. Neurogenic duplication cyst.

Q. 54
Which of the following mediastinal lesions in relation to others presents with paraplegia?

A. Bronchogenic cyst.
B. Neurogenic duplication cyst.
C. Neuroblastoma.
D. Neratoma.
E. Thymic hyperplasia.

Q. 55
Neuroblastoma which is localised primary tumour with dissemination limited to skin, liver, and/or bone marrow in infants younger than 1 year of age is labelled as:

A. Stage I.
B. Stage II.
C. Stage III.
D. Stage IV.
E. Stage IV-S.

Q. 56
Common effects of neuroblastoma on kidneys are:

A. Dilatation.
B. Displacement.
C. Distortion.
D. All of the above.
E. None of the above.

Bone Tumour

Q. 57
Sunburst appearance is a radiological feature of which of the following tumours?

- A. Pheochromocytoma.
- B. Ewing Sarcoma.
- C. Teratoma
- D. Osteosarcoma.
- E. Neuroblastoma.

Testicular Tumour

Q. 58
Regarding testicular tumours, which of the following is false?

- A. Testicular tumours account for 1 percent of tumours in children.
- B. Teratoma is mostly benign.
- C. Most common malignant tumour is germ cell tumour.
- D. Sertoli cell tumour causes gynaecomastia.
- E. Seminoma is the most common tumour.

Q. 59
Microscopic residual tumour is a feature of which stage of testicular tumour.

- A. Stage I.
- B. Stage II.
- C. Stage III.
- D. Stage IV.
- E. None of the above.

Q. 60
Regarding testicular tumour marker, which of the following statements is not true?

A. Alpha-fetoprotein and beta-HCG both are glycoprotein.
B. Alpha-fetoprotein half-life is 5 days.
C. Beta HCG half-life is 24 hours.
D. Alpha-fetoprotein level comes to normal after 2 days of surgery.
E. B-HCG level comes to normal after 5–7 days of surgery.

Q. 61
A Tumour that develops from the dysgenetic gonad is:

A. Yolk sac tumour.
B. Teratoma.
C. Gonadoblastoma.
D. Leiomyoma.
E. Seminoma.

Q. 62
Which of the following is not germ cell tumour?

A. Leydig cell.
B. Yolk sac.
C. Mixed germ cell tumour.
D. Seminoma.
E. Teratoma.

SECTION 11

VESSELS AND LYMPHATICS

Vascular Malformation

Q. 1
Regarding arteriovenous malformation, which of the following is false?

   A. Most occur in peripheral vessels.
   B. Macro fistulous are obvious and easily seen on angiography.
   C. Mostly seen in lower limbs.
   D. Can be classified as micro-fistulous and macro-fistulous.
   E. May be associated with hemi-atrophy of limb.

Q. 2
Regarding congenital aneurysm, which one of the following is false?

   A. Usually involves visceral arteries.
   B. Rupture is unusual.

C. Hypotension is common when renal artery branches are involved.
D. Common in spleen and liver.
E. Repair is indicated for more than 2 cm.

Q. 3
Features of midaortic syndrome include all except:

A. Fibromuscular dysplasia.
B. Aortic aneurysm.
C. Malignant hypertension.
D. Congestive cardiac failure.
E. Renal failure.

Q. 4
Regarding Klippel-Trenaunay syndrome, all of the following are correct except:

A. Limb hypertrophy.
B. Lymphatic dysplasia.
C. Port wine stain.
D. Venous hypertension.
E. Varicose vein.

Q. 5
The following are diffuse congenital malformations of venous predominance except:

A. Haemangioma.
B. Klippel-Trenaunay syndrome.
C. Proteus syndrome.
D. Parkes-Weber syndrome.
E. Maffucci syndrome.

Q. 6
About arteriovenous malformation all of the following are correct except:

A. Usually slow flow.
B. Present at birth.
C. Evident on infancy.
D. Skin becomes red or violaceous.
E. Local warmth, thrill or bruit.

Q. 7
The best sclerosing agent used to manage lymphatic malformation is:

A. One hundred per cent ethanol.
B. Sodium tetradecyl sulphate.
C. Bleomycin.
D. OK432.
E. Any of the above.

Q. 8
What is false about haemangioma?

A. They are tumours of vascular tissue.
B. They are the third most common soft tumour of infancy.
C. They are the most common congenital anomaly in humans.
D. Incidence is 1–3 percent.
E. Female to male ratio 3:1.

Q. 9
The following are variety of capillary haemangioma except:

- A. Salmon pink.
- B. Strawberry nevus.
- C. Port wine stain.
- D. Spider nevus.
- E. Cystic hygroma.

Q. 10
Regarding management of haemangioma, which is false?

- A. About 25 percent naturally undergo involution.
- B. Corticosteroid is one method of treatment.
- C. Alpha interferon is used for serious and life-threatening haemangioma.
- D. Laser therapy is only used in cutaneous haemangioma.
- E. Excision should be performed in involution phase.

Lymphatic Malformation

Q. 11
Which of the following is not true about lymphangioma?

- A. Majority apparent at birth.
- B. OK432 is helpful in treatment.
- C. Mortality in general is less than 10 percent.
- D. Intrathoracic has higher mortality than cervicomediastinal.
- E. Lymphangioma of extremities has low mortality.

Q. 12
Regarding lymphatic disorders, all of the following are false except:

A. Fluid in chylothorax contains more than 20 percent of lymphocytes.
B. Cavernous lymphangioma comprises of capillary-sized lymphatic channels.
C. Cystic hygroma undergoes malignancy.
D. Bleomycin is one of the treatment of lymphangioma.
E. In chylous ascites, internal drainage by percutaneous shunt is not possible.

Q. 13
Regarding lymphedema, which statement is false?

A. There is increase lymph in interstitial tissue.
B. Primary lymphedema is more common than secondary.
C. Lymphedema Praecox is secondary type of lymphedema.
D. Lymphedema Tarda presents after 35 years of age.
E. Excision surgery by Charles method involves removal of skin and subcutaneous tissues down to the muscle and covering the nude surface with split-thickness skin graft.

Q. 14
Regarding cystic hygroma, all of the following are correct except:

A. It is lined by endothelial cells.
B. It is a cluster of lymphatic channels that fails to connect to normal lymphatic pathway.
C. Fifty to seventy per cent appear one month after birth.
D. It appears as lump at lower third of neck.
E. Cystic lymphangioma is same as cystic hygroma.

Q. 15
The following are the slow flow vascular malformation except:

A. Telangiectasia.
B. Klippel-Trenaunay syndrome.
C. Proteus syndrome.
D. Solomon syndrome.
E. Parkes-Weber syndrome.

Q. 16
Vascular malformation is different from haemangioma by all of the following features except:

A. It is a developmental error of vessels.
B. It is composed of dysplastic vessels.
C. It almost never regresses.
D. It is present at birth.
E. It is marked by ulceration and bleeding.

SECTION 12

ANATOMY FOR PAEDIATRIC SURGEONS

Thorax

Q. 1
Regarding the development of diaphragm, which of the following statements is true?

A. Receives contribution from body wall.
B. Receives contribution from ventral mesentery.
C. Formed mainly from septum transverse.
D. Receives contribution from pleuroperitoneal membrane.
E. Receives contribution from dorsal mesentery of intestine.

Q. 2
Regarding structures passing through the diaphragm, which is not true?

A. Oesophageal opening is surrounded by left crus of diaphragm.
B. The splanchnic nerve pierces the crura.
C. The sympathetic nerves passes behind medial arcuate ligament.
D. The left phrenic nerve pierces the left dome of diaphragm.
E. The anterior and posterior gastric nerves transmitted with the oesophagus.

Q. 3
Regarding azygos vein, which of the following is true?

A. Originates in the abdomen.
B. Leaves through oesophageal opening.
C. Drains in the right atrium directly.
D. Drains left intercostal and bronchial vein directly.
E. Does not receive the hemi-azygos vein.

Q. 4
Regarding the right vagus nerve, what is false?

A. Lies posterolateral to right brachiocephalic artery.
B. Lies between trachea and mediastinum.
C. Lives branches to pulmonary plexus.
D. Gives branches to oesophageal plexus.
E. Changes its name as posterior gastric nerve.

Q. 5
Regarding the thymus, which of the following is true?

    A. Atrophied shortly after birth.
    B. Lies posterior to trachea.
    C. Derived from fourth pair of pharyngeal pouch.
    D. Has cortex and medulla.
    E. Contains mainly monocytes.

Q. 6
Regarding thoracic oesophagus, which of the following is false?

    A. Lies posterior to trachea.
    B. Related to left atrium.
    C. Oesophageal opening in diaphragm is left of midline.
    D. Oesophageal opening is at the level of 8th thoracic vertebrae.
    E. Directly related to vertebral column in its upper part.

Q. 7
Regarding thoracic trachea, which of the following statements is false?

    A. It has complete rings.
    B. Rings are made up of hyaline cartilage.
    C. Bifurcation is at the level of fourth thoracic vertebrae.
    D. It is closely related to azygos vein.
    E. Thymus gland is found in front of trachea.

Q. 8
Regarding right lung, which of the following statements is false?

A. It is larger than left.
B. Possess ten bronchopulmonary segments.
C. It is divided by fissures into upper and lower lobes and lingual.
D. It is related to the oesophagus in most of its thoracic course.
E. Lung segments are more than left lung.

Q. 9
Regarding thoracic duct, which of the following statements is false?

A. Ascends anterior to vertebral column.
B. Arises in thorax.
C. Drains in left broncho-cephalic vein.
D. Drains all the body below the diaphragm and left half of the body above the diaphragm.
E. Arises from cisterna chyli.

Abdomen

Q. 10
At birth, the umbilical cord contains none of the following except:

A. Patent urachus.
B. Patent vitellointestinal duct.
C. Patent umbilical arteries and vein.
D. Patent right umbilical vein.
E. Patent two umbilical veins and two arteries.

Q. 11
Regarding lateral muscles of anterior abdominal wall, which statement is false?

A. It is attached in part to the costal cartilage.
B. It is supplied by lower six thoracic and first lumbar nerve.
C. It is attached to lateral margin of rectus abdominis.
D. Rectus sheath is formed by the aponeurosis of three lateral muscles.
E. The aponeurosis of internal oblique splits to enclose rectus abdominis in the umbilical region.

Q. 12
Regarding the inguinal canal, which of the following statements is false?

A. Deep inguinal ring is a defect in fascia transversalis laterally.
B. Superficial inguinal ring is a defect in the external oblique aponeurosis medially.
C. Has anterior wall comprising the external oblique aponeurosis and internal oblique muscle.
D. The floor is the upper surface of the inguinal ligament.
E. Posterior wall is formed medially by peritoneum only.

Q. 13
Regarding spermatic cord, which of the following statements is false?

A. Has three fascial coverings.
B. Contains three arteries.
C. Contains three nerves.

D. Contains one muscle.
E. Contains three veins.

Q. 14
Regarding the testes, which of the following statements is false?

A. The epididymis is at the posterolateral aspect.
B. Lymphatic drainage is to external iliac lymph nodes.
C. It descends in the scrotum just before birth.
D. Is supplied by sympathetic nerves, originating from tenth thoracic segment.
E. It takes covering of peritoneum, the processus vaginalis while descend.

Q. 15
Regarding the development of the testes, which statement is false?

A. It develops from colonic mesothelium of posterior abdominal wall.
B. The tubules of mesonephric become the efferent duct and the head of epididymis.
C. The mesonephric duct becomes ductus deference.
D. Testicular descent is aided by gubernaculum.
E. It originates from metanephros.

Q. 16
Regarding lesser omentum, which of the following statements is false?

A. It is attached superiorly with to the porta hepatitis and fissure for ligamentum venosum.
B. It extends inferiorly as for as transverse colon.

C. It lies behind lesser sac and stomach.
D. It communicates with the greater sac only by the epiploic foramen.
E. It forms part of boundaries of the epiploic foramen.

Q. 17
Regarding mesentery, which of the following statements is false?

A. Its oblique attachment extends from the duodenojejunal flexure (on the left side of the L2 vertebrae to the ileocecal junction, overlying the sacroiliac joint).
B. The arteries it contains are branches of superior mesenteric artery.
C. Its horizontal attachment extends to the left across the descending part of the duodenum, the anterior border of the pancreases, and the tail of pancreas as it crosses the anterior surface of the left kidney.
D. Mesentery of sigmoid colon lies over promontory of sacrum.
E. The arteries it contains supply the midgut.

Q. 18
Regarding abdominal oesophagus, which statement is false?

A. It is enveloped by the peritoneum.
B. The oesophageal opening in the diaphragm lies within the fibres of right crus to the left of the midline.
C. It is closely related with the anterior and posterior gastric nerves.
D. It is closely related to the left lobe of the liver.
E. Intra-abdominal oesophagus is important to prevent gastroesophageal reflux.

Q. 19
Regarding the stomach, which of the following statements is false?

A. It is partly supplied by arteries arising from splenic artery.
B. It is lined by columnar and squamous epithelium.
C. All blood from the stomach normally passes normally passes through the portal vein.
D. It is supplied by arteries that arise from branches of coeliac trunk.
E. It contains three types of glands.

Q. 20
Regarding the duodenum, which of the following statements is false?

A. Lies anterior to hilum of right kidney.
B. Crosses anteriorly by superior mesenteric vessels.
C. Lies behind portal vein.
D. Only first and last centimetre are invested by peritoneum.
E. Only anterior surface is covered by peritoneum.

Q. 21
Regarding the small intestine, which of the following is false?

A. Jejunum has thicker wall than ileum.
B. Atrial arcades are less numerous in jejunum than ileum.
C. Root of mesentery crosses the left psoas muscle.
D. Duodenojejunal flexure lies on left of first lumbar vertebrae.
E. Jejunum has wider than ileum.

Q. 22
Regarding the caecum, which of the following statements is false?

A. It is completely invested in the peritoneum.
B. It lies on the right psoas muscle.
C. The longitudinal muscles are arranged in three bands.
D. The muscle bands of caecum converge on the appendix.
E. It has ileocecal orifice opening inferiorly.

Q. 23
Regarding the appendix, which statement is false?

A. It has a mesentery.
B. It usually lies retrocaecally.
C. It arises from the posteromedial wall of caecum, 3 cm below the ileocecal valve.
D. Absence of appendix is extremely rare.
E. Its length is the same in all children.

Q. 24
Regarding celiac trunk, which of the following statements is false?

A. Superior mesenteric artery is its branch.
B. It arises from the aorta just above the pancreas.
C. It has three main branches.
D. It is surrounded by plexus of nerves.
E. It supplies to the foregut and structures derived from it.

Q. 25
Regarding splenic artery which one of the following statements is false?

A. It supplies branches to the left adrenal gland.
B. Its initial course along upper border of pancreas is retroperitoneal.
C. It reaches at hilum of spleen through splenorenal ligament.
D. Its short gastric branches passes through gastro-splenic ligament.
E. Its left gastroepiploic branch passes to greater curvature of stomach.

Q. 26
Portosystemic anastomosis occurs in all of the following sites except:

A. Azygos vein and left gastric vein.
B. Epigastric vein and vein in falciform ligament.
C. Anorectal junction.
D. Bar area of gut, liver and pancreas.
E. Portal vein and renal vein.

Q. 27
Regarding the anatomy of the liver, which of the following is false?

A. It divides into two lobes on the visceral surface by interloper fissure.
B. Liver has a fibrous capsule.
C. It is totally covered by peritoneum.

D. It is attached by falciform ligament to anterior abdominal wall and diaphragm.
E. It is attached with inferior vena cava.

Q. 28
Regarding liver anatomy, all of the following are true except:

A. It drains by hepatic vein into inferior vena cava.
B. It has lymph drainage to both mediastinal and porto hepatic nodes.
C. It is supplied by branches from both vagus nerve.
D. It is directly related to right supra-renal gland.
E. Parasympathetic fibres are supplied through coeliac plexus.

Q. 29
Regarding the bile duct, which one of the following statements is false?

A. It enters the duodenum at its medial wall.
B. Behind the first part of duodenum, it lies anterior to the portal vein.
C. Behind the head of the pancreas, it lies anterior to the inferior vena cava.
D. It joins the main pancreatic duct to open in to the ampulla.
E. It enters the duodenum 20 cm from the pylorus.

Q. 30
Regarding the gallbladder, which of the following statements is false?

A. It is closely related to the duodenum.

B. Its fundus is in contact with the anterior abdominal wall, deep to the tip of the ninth costal cartilage.
C. It is supplied by the cystic artery, a branch of the right hepatic artery.
D. It is lined by squamous epithelium.
E. It contains mucus-secreting goblet cells.

Q. 31
Regarding the spleen, all of the following are true except:

A. Its anterior surface is directly related to lesser curvature of stomach.
B. It lies deep to left 9th, 10th and 11th ribs.
C. It is separated from the chest wall by the diaphragm.
D. The tail of the pancreases extends into the lienorenal ligament.
E. Arterial supply is from the coeliac trunk.

Q. 32
Regarding the anatomy of the pancreas, all of the following are true except:

A. Both renal vein joins the inferior vena cava, behind the head of the pancreas.
B. It is related to both the greater sac of peritoneum and the omental bursa.
C. It usually has two major ducts.
D. It is completely invested in the peritoneum.
E. Transverse mesocolon is attached to the anterior border.

Pelvis

Q. 33
Regarding the sacrum, all of the following are true except:

A. It is made up of four vertebrae.
B. It has foramina communicating with central canal.
C. Poor development may lead to faecal incontinence.
D. The association of imperforate anus and sacral agenesis is well known.
E. It gives attachment to erector spinae muscle.

Q. 34
Regarding levator ani muscle, which of the following is false?

A. It is supplied largely by sympathetic and parasympathetic nerves.
B. The anterior fibres pass around the urethra and prostate (urethra and vagina in female) to the fibrous perineal body.
C. Its middle fibres pass medially around the rectum to the anococcygeal body.
D. The posterior fibres pass to the midline raphe and the coccyx.
E. It provides muscular support to the pelvic viscera and reinforces the rectal and urethral sphincter.

Q. 35
Regarding the anatomy of the rectum, all of the following are true except:

A. It begins in front of the third sacral vertebrae.
B. It has no mesentery.

C. It has venous drainage to superior mesenteric vein.
D. Lymphatic drainage passes along the superior rectal vessels to the para-aortic and laterally to the internal iliac nodes.
E. It is lined by columnar epithelium.

Q. 36
Regarding the anatomy of the anal canal, which of the following is false?

A. The internal sphincter is involuntary.
B. The internal sphincter is continuous with circular muscle of rectum.
C. The external sphincter encircles the lower two-thirds of the anal canal.
D. The external sphincter has deep, superficial, and subcutaneous parts.
E. The external sphincter is supplied by parasympathetic nerves.

Q. 37
Regarding the anatomy of the urinary bladder, which of the following is false?

A. It is attached to the umbilicus.
B. It has no peritoneal covering.
C. It is largely supported by pelvic fascia.
D. It has sensory supply by both sympathetic and parasympathetic system.
E. Sympathetic fibres are motor to vesical sphincter and parasympathetic fibres e motor to bladder wall.

Q. 38
Regarding the broad ligament of the uterus, which of the following statements is false?

A. The broad ligament extends from the lateral pelvic wall to the lateral margin of the uterus.
B. Uterine arteries lie in the medial two-thirds of its upper border.
C. Suspensory ligament of the ovary lies in the lateral one-third of free upper border of broad ligament and contains ovarian vessels.
D. It contains the round ligament of uterus.
E. It extends to the inguinal canal.

Q. 39
Regarding ovaries, which of the following statements is false?

A. Has lymphatic drainage to the internal iliac lymph node.
B. Receives blood supply from branches of uterine arteries.
C. Is related on its lateral surface to the uterine tube.
D. Lies on the back of broad ligament.
E. Ovarian arteries arise from aorta.

Q. 40
Regarding ductus deferens, which of the following statements is false?

A. It is continuation of canal/tail of epididymis.
B. It joins the duct of seminal vesical to form ejaculatory duct.
C. It ends by opening in prostatic urethra.

D. It lies medial to seminal vesical.
E. Terminal part descends posterior to the bladder.

Q. 41
Regarding the anatomy of the penis, which one of the following statements is false?

A. It comprises the cylinders of erectile tissues.
B. The ventral corpus spongiosum expands anteriorly to forms the glans penis.
C. The corpus cavernous diverges posteriorly to form the crura of the penis.
D. The bulb of the penis is formed by the corpus spongiosum posteriorly.
E. It has lymphatic drainage to the internal iliac lymph nodes.

Q. 42
Regarding the anatomy of the male urethra, which of the following statements is false?

A. Receives midline ejaculatory duct.
B. Receives 20–30 prostatic ducts.
C. Traverses the whole length of corpus spongiosum.
D. Has the sphincter urethra muscle surrounds its membranous part.
E. Sphincter urethra lies between prostate and the bulb.

Q. 43
Regarding the pudendal nerve, which of the following statements is false?

A. Arises from lumbar plexus.

B. Supplies levator ani.
C. Supplies perineal skin.
D. Supplies external anal sphincter.
E. Supplies urethral sphincter.

Q. 44
Regarding the cisterna chyli, which of the following statements is false?

A. Drains directly into the left jugular vein.
B. Lies between right crus of diaphragm and aorta.
C. Receives right and left lumbar lymphatic trunk.
D. Receives from abdominal alimentary tract.
E. Leads directly into the thoracic duct.

Q. 45
External anal sphincter is supplied by:

A. Sympathetic.
B. Parasympathetic.
C. L1 and L2.
D. L3 and L4.
E. S2 to S4.

Urogenital System

Q. 46
Which of the following is true regarding the development of external genitalia?

A. Genital folds form the labia minora.
B. Cloacal swelling forms the glans penis.

C. Laterally placed cloacal membrane develops into the body of penis.
D. Cloacal swelling forms labia minora in females.
E. Genital tubercle forms the clitoris in females.

Q. 47
Regarding kidneys, which one of the following is false?

A. The hila lies close to the trans-pyloric plan, at the level of the second lumbar vertebrae.
B. The diaphragm separates them from eleventh and twelfth rib.
C. They lie in the fascial sheath with their related suprarenal gland.
D. At the hilum of each kidney, the renal vein, artery, and pelvis of ureter lie in the order of front to back.
E. Secreting part of kidney develops from metanephros.

Q. 48
Regarding the ureter, which of the following statements is false?

A. Ureteric course in the pelvis is the same in each sex.
B. Both ureters descend on psoas.
C. Ureter crosses the bifurcation of common iliac vessels in front of the sacroiliac joint.
D. Ductus deferens crosses the ureters in males.
E. In females, ureters are crossed over by uterine arteries.

Q. 49
Regarding the suprarenal gland, which of the following is false?

A. The right gland is pyramidal in shape, while the left is crescentic in shape.
B. Receives branches from thoracic sympathetic trunk through splanchnic nerves.
C. Preganglionic fibres end in medulla of the gland.
D. On each side is related to inferior vena cava.
E. Both have rich blood supply.

Q. 50
Regarding renal arteries, which of the following statements is false?

A. Left renal artery is shorter.
B. Renal arteries arise from aorta at the level of second lumbar vertebrae.
C. Both are related to the crus of the diaphragm on the same side.
D. It supplies branches to the corresponding suprarenal gland and ureter.
E. It gives testicular (or ovarian) branches.

Q. 51
Regarding inferior vena cava, which of the following statements is false?

A. Caval opening lies in the central tendon of the diaphragm to the right of mid-line.
B. Receives tributaries from both gonadal veins.
C. Receives several hepatic veins.

D. Formed in front of fifth lumbar vertebrae.
E. Hepatic veins enter the part of vena cava, which usually enters in the liver.

Limbs

Q. 52
Regarding the epiphysis of bones, which one of the following statements is false?

A. They are secondary centres of ossification.
B. These are presents in all long bones.
C. Formed by osteoblasts.
D. Increases the girth of long bones.
E. Only those of the knee presents at birth.

Q. 53
Regarding the anatomy of the axilla, which of the following statements is false?

A. Posterior wall is formed by the subscapularis.
B. Serratus anterior forms medial boundary.
C. Apex is bounded by medial third of clavicle.
D. Apex is communicated with posterior triangle of neck.
E. Anterior wall is formed by pectoralis major.

Q. 54
Regarding the brachial plexus, which of the following statements is false?

A. It is usually formed by the ventral rami of the lower four cervical and first thoracic nerve.
B. Contains three trunks, which lies in the neck.

C. Upper two roots form the upper trunk, middle root continues as the middle trunk, and the lower two form the lower trunk.
D. Cords are formed in the apex of the axilla behind the middle third of the clavicle.
E. Cords are named according to their arrangement around the subclavian artery.

Q. 55
Regarding cubital fossa, which of the following statements is false?

A. It is quadrangular spaced in front of the elbow joint.
B. Bicipital aponeurosis forms the roof.
C. Contains from medial to lateral, median nerve, brachial artery, biceps tendon, radial nerve, and posterior interosseous nerve.
D. Bounded proximally by a line joining two epicondyle of humorous.
E. Bounded distally by pronator teres medially and brachioradialis laterally.

Q. 56
Regarding femoral triangle, which of the following is false?

A. The arrangement of vein, artery and nerve from medial to lateral respectively.
B. The femoral vein separated by femoral canal from lacunar part of inguinal ligament.
C. It is bounded medially by the adductor longus muscle.
D. The femoral artery forms behind the midpoint of the inguinal ligament.

E. The triangle has a defect in the fascial roof for greater saphenous vein.

Q. 57
Regarding popliteal vessels, which of the following statements is false?

A. Popliteal artery is deep to popliteal vein and tibial nerve.
B. Popliteal vein is deep to tibial nerve.
C. Popliteal artery is superficial to popliteal vein.
D. Both popliteal artery and vein are deep to tibial nerve.
E. Popliteal artery lies deep on the lower posterior surface of femur.

Q. 58
Regarding the great saphenous vein, which of the following is true?

A. Passes behind medial malleolus.
B. Enters femoral vein in the middle of thigh.
C. Usually receives blood from deep vein in the thigh.
D. Accompanies saphenous nerve in the leg.
E. Joins external iliac vein.

Head and Neck

Q. 59
Regarding superior aspect of skull, which of the following statements is false?

A. Coronal sutures separate the frontal from parietal bone.
B. Lambda (posterior fontanelle) lies between sagittal and lambdoid sutures.

C. Bregma (anterior fontanelle) is between sagittal, coronal, and frontal sutures.
D. Posterior fontanelle is usually closed by second to third month after birth.
E. Anterior fontanelle is closed by about six months after birth.

Q. 60
Regarding muscles and movement of eyeball, which of the following statements is false?

A. Inferior rectus is supplied by inferior division of oculomotor nerve.
B. Superior rectus is supplied by upper division of oculomotor nerve.
C. Lateral rectus is supplied by lateral division of trochlear nerve.
D. Downward and lateral movement is by superior oblique.
E. Superior oblique is supplied by trochlear nerve.

Q. 61
Regarding deciduous teeth, which of the following statements is false?

A. First lower incisor tooth erupts at one year of age.
B. First permanent teeth appear at six years of age.
C. The lower permanent teeth appear slightly earlier.
D. There are no deciduous premolar teeth.
E. Derive their denture from mesenchyme.

Q. 62
Regarding the palate, which of the following statements is false?

A. In the hard palate, incisive foramen transmits lesser palatine artery.
B. Palatine process for hard palate develops from maxillary process.
C. Soft palate has different form of epithelium at its upper and lower surface.
D. Tensor vali palatine tendon forms aponeurosis of soft palate.
E. Vagus nerve innervates all the muscles of palate except tensor vali palatine through the pharyngeal plexus.

Q. 63
Regarding the gland, which of the following statements is false?

A. In the parotid gland, external carotid artery is deep to the fascial nerve within its substance.
B. Submandibular gland and sublingual glands are mixed glands, while parotid gland is serous gland.
C. Sublingual gland partly secretes into the submandibular duct.
D. Submandibular duct opens at the level of upper second molar teeth.
E. Parasympathetic fibres for parotid glands are from nasopharyngeal nerve.

Q. 64
Regarding the boundaries of the posterior triangle of the neck, which of the following statements is false?

A. It is bordered anteriorly by sternocleidomastoid muscle.
B. Posterior border is formed by rhomboids major muscle.
C. Middle third of clavicle forms inferior border.
D. Floor is formed by prevertebral fascia with overlying muscles.
E. It is not divided into further triangles like the anterior triangle of neck.

Vertebral Column

Q. 65
Regarding vertebral column, which of the following statements is false?

A. C1 has no spine.
B. C7 is called vertebral prominence.
C. Radiograph of allanto-occipital joint are taken by open mouth.
D. There is intervertebral disc between C1 and C2.
E. Primary foetal curvature is retained in thoracic and sacral region.

Q. 66
Regarding the vertebral column, which of the following statements is false?

A. Dura covering spinal cord fuses with the periosteum of adjacent vertebrae.
B. Spinal cord ends at L2.

C. In lower part of canal, the nerves run with increasing obliquity before emerging in through foramina.
D. Dorsal root ganglion is situated near the point of fusion of nerve roots.
E. Internal vertebral veins have large branches draining the bodies of vertebrae.

ANSWERS

Section 1

ABOMEN- A

PYLORIC STENOSIS

Ans.1
B
Pyloric stenosis.
All features in question are suggestive of pyloric stenosis.

Ans.2
A
The pyloric muscle thickness 4 mm or more and pyloric channel length 16 mm or more.

Ans.3
A
Anterosuperior surface.
This is relatively bloodless area.

Ans.4
D
Hypochloremic, hypokalemic metabolic alkalosis. Hypochloraemia because of loss of chloride in vomitus. Hypokalaemia because of K^+ loss in vomitus and activation of rennin-AG-ALD system will produce loss of K^+ in urine. With K^+ loss in urine, it gets reabsorbed in distal tubule with loss of H^+ worsening, leading to metabolic alkalosis and production of acidic urine. Initially, alkaline urine and, later, paradoxical aciduria is noted, in order to prevent hypokalaemia. Metabolic alkalosis also because of loss of H^+ in vomitus, decreased secretion of pancreatic CHO_3^-, increased CHO_3^- presented to distal tubule and eliminated, producing an alkaline urine.

Additionally, hyponatraemia occurs because of loss of Na^+ in vomitus, decreased absorption of Na^+, and loss of Na^+ in urine until kidney adjusts to increased CHO_3^- load.

DUODENAL ATRESIA

Ans.5
C
Duodenal atresia.
The conditions most likely associated with duodenal atresia are Down syndrome, malrotation, congenital heart disease, annular pancreas and oesophageal atresia.

Ans.6
E
Blind ends of duodenum connected with fibrous cord.

Ans.7
D
If trans-anastomotic tube is placed, immediate enteral feed can be started.

Ans.8
B
Leaving small part on medial side is intact because of chance of damage of ampulla of Vater.

D and E are preferred method of for type II and type III atresia.

Ans.9
E
All of the above are true.

Ans.10
C
Windsock is a variant of type I atresia. Type I atresia is the commonest. Obstruction below the ampulla is seen in 85 per cent of cases. Survival rate is 90–95 percent. Most deaths are due to complex congenital heart disease.

JEJUNAL ATRESIA/ILEAL ATRESIA

Ans.11
C
Jaundice is common in jejunal atresia.

Ans.12
D
Type III B atresia is called apple peel variety of jejunal atresia.

223

MECONIUM ILEUS

Ans.13
D
Cystic fibrosis is one of the causes of meconium ileus, not the complication.

Ans.14
D
Microcolon is a feature on contrast enema.

Ans.15
E
All of the above.

Ans.16
A
Gastrographin leads to diarrhoea.

Ans.17
E
All of the above have been seen in children with meconium ileus. Other complications include appendicitis, rectal prolapse, colonic stricture, cholelithiasis, hydrocele, undescended testes and absence of vas deference.

Ans.18
B
Disorder involving chromosome number 7.

Ans.19
E
Pancreatic insufficiency is seen in 90 percent of cases, meconium ileus in about 20 percent of cases, obstructive biliary diseases in about 15 percent of cases, and azoospermia in nearly all of affected males.

Ans.20
A
>90 percent

Ans.21
C
Meconium ileus with early gestational age, perforation leads to Meconium cyst formation.

On plain X-rays, it shows calcification with air-fluid level.

Ans.22
D
80 per cent.

Ans.23
D
A and B are true.

MALROTATION

Ans.24
E
Rotation occurs between tenth and twelfth weeks of gestation.

Ans.25
A
Dilatation of either small intestinal loop or only stomach and duodenum is a feature of mal-rotation, not the colon.

Ans.26
C
In Ladd's procedure, one should take care of superior mesenteric artery.

An additional step in Ladd's procedure is the placement of caecum in left hypochondrium.

Ans.27
E
Meconium ileus has different pathology.

Ans.28
A
Normal intestinal rotation involves 270-degree counterclockwise rotation of duodenojejunal loop around the superior mesenteric artery.

Ans.29
D
All of the above are correct.

Ans.30
E
Regarding the procedure for malrotation, all mentioned are different steps.

Ans.31
B
Between 4–10 weeks of gestational age.

ACHALASIA CARDIA

Ans.32
B
Histochemistry shows decrease, not increase, in neuropeptide, VIP and gastrin.

Ans.33
D
Barium meal shows narrowing of lower oesophagus. CT is not the investigation of choice, plain X-rays may shows air-fluid level in lower oesophagus. Barium meal shows rate tail appearance due to funnelling and narrowing of oesophagus. 24- hours pH monitoring is required for diagnosis of gastroesophageal reflux.

Ans.34
E
Loose (floppy) fundoplication is part of the procedure.

Ans.35
E
Gastroesophageal reflux incidence is about 15 percent, while residual or recurrence is 25 per cent.

INTUSSUSCEPTION

Ans.36
B
The A, C and D possible, but most likely diagnosis is intussusception.

Ans.37
E
Pressure required is 80–150 mm Hg. Initial part reduces rapidly. Quite often, intussusception lodges in caecum for that sustained pressure of for 3–4 minutes is required. Benchmark of reduction is reflux of contrast or gas in different loops of ileum. Ultrasound shows target sign on transverse image and pseudo kidney sign on longitudinal image.

Ans.38
C
Resection is necessary if necrotic bowel.

Ans.39
B
About 10 percent recurrence rate noted after pneumatic reduction.

Ans.40
E
All statements A, B and C are true. Other suspected causes may include change in diet, misappropriate size between ileum and ileocolic valve, Meckel's diverticulum, polyp, neuro fibroma, haemangioma, hypertrophied lymphoid patch, submucosal haematoma, lymphoma, abdominal trauma and various surgical procedures.

VITELLOINTESTINAL DUCT ANOMALIES

Ans.41
E
Ectopic gastric mucosa presents with melena, bands presents with intestinal obstruction. Meckel's diverticulum that leads to intussusception, presents with abdominal pain, mass, and red currant jelly in stool. Patent vitellointestinal duct presents with passage of air and faeces from umbilicus. Shiny, spherical red nodule is a feature of umbilical polyp (ectopic mucosa at umbilicus). Meckel's diverticulitis presents with abdominal pain, vomiting, and fever. On examination, tenderness in right lower abdomen. These features are the same as appendicitis.

Ans.42
A
Blood is noted in umbilical polyp and urine is seen in patent urachus.

Ans.43
D
Skin incision depends upon features and type of presentation. When vitellointestinal duct anomaly presents with feature of band or intussusception, supra-umbilical transverse incision is preferred. When presents with features of diverticulitis or ectopic gastric mucosa (melena), infra-umbilical incision is preferred. When presents with patent vitellointestinal duct (fistula) then make an incision at the level of the umbilicus or an infra-umbilical curved incision.

Ans. 44
A
Urachus connects bladder to allantois. Omphalomesenteric duct connects mid-gut to yolk sac.

Ans.45
B
Lateral umbilical ligament is remnant of umbilical arteries.

Ans.46
E
All of the above mentioned are uses of umbilicus.

Ans.47
C
Meckel's diverticulum is the most common anomaly of GIT caused by failure of regression of vitellin duct. The rich blood supply to the diverticulum is provided by the vitelline artery, which is a branch of the superior mesenteric artery. Among heterotopic mucosa, gastric mucosa is more commonly found than pancreatic mucosa. If Meckel's diverticulum goes in hernia sac, it is called Litter's hernia.

Ans.48
C
Meckel's diverticulum is usually located within two feet of ileocecal valve.

Ans.49
C
Glucagon, pentagastrin, and histamine blockers increase the accuracy of scanning. False positive results may be due to

duplication cyst, gastro-genic cyst, ulcers, inflammatory bowel disease, bowel obstruction and neoplasm.

Ans.50
E
If left intact the lifetime risk of complication of Meckel's diverticulum is 6.4 percent.

OMPHALOCELE AND GASTROSCHISIS

Ans.51
E
Silver sulfadiazine is safer compared to other agents used in eschar formation.

Ans.52
A
Omphalocele minor is defined as small defect and hernial contents are usually a few loops of small intestine. Reduction of content and primary repair is the best option.

Ans.53
B
It occurs at the level of umbilicus. The umbilical cord is attached at the apex of sac.

Ans.54
A
Primary closure is ideal option among mentioned options. In addition to above-mentioned options, other options include amnion inversion, coverage of the intact sac with Eschar-inducing agent.

Ans.55
E
Malrotation is present in both. The omphalocele is attached at umbilical ring and gastroschisis is present right to umbilical ring. In omphalocele, defect is variable (4–10 cm), sac is present or ruptured and cord is attached on to the base. In gastroschisis, size of defect is <4 cm, sac is absent and cord is attached at normal position.

Ans.56
A
Involution of right umbilical vein leads to development of gastroschisis.

Ans.57
E
Generally, vitamin K is required prophylactically to achieve good haemostasis at the time of surgery. Other immediate management techniques include avoiding hypothermia, as well as correcting electrolytes, calcium, glucose, FBC, ABG and prophylactic antibiotics.

Ans.58
C
Silver nitrate 0.5 per cent solution is used, not 10 percent.

Ans.59
C
Necrotizing enterocolitis is early or immediate complication of gastroschisis.

Ans.60
B
Complete primary closure in gastroschisis can be performed in more than 60 percent of cases.

Ans.61
D
All mentioned are true.

Ans.62
D
Adhesion formation makes volvulus very rare event after gastroschisis repair.

Ans.63
D
Tetralogy of Fallot.

Ans.64
A
The defect is to the right of umbilicus.

ASCITIES

Ans.65
A
Congenital hepatic fibrosis does not causes biliary ascites. It causes hepatocellular variety of ascites. Other causes of biliary ascites include spontaneous perforation of bile duct, congenital weakness of bile duct and localised mural malformation of wall of common bile duct.

Ans.66
E
Atresia or stenosis of major lacteal at base of mesentery or cisterna chyli leads to chylous ascites. Other causes of hepatocellular ascites include viral hepatitis, neonatal hepatitis and congenital hepatic fibrosis.

Ans.67
C
Albumin level in ascitic fluid in urinary ascites is <50 mg per 100 ml.

Ans.68
D
Peritoneovenous catheter is an option in chylous and hepatocellular ascites, not in urinary ascites.

TRICHOBEZOAR

Ans.69
E
Collection of hairs in the stomach by ingestion is called trichobezoar. Phytobezoar is made up of vegetable fibres and pharmacobezoar is from medications.

Section 2

ABDOMEN B

PANCREAS

Ans.1
E
Dorsal bud forms most of pancreas. Normally, ventral bud rotates backward; if it does not occur, the condition is called annular pancreas. Normally duct of Wirsung becomes the major duct in the end. If two-duct system fails to fuse, condition is called pancreatic divisum. In this condition, dorsal duct (duct of Santorini) becomes the main duct. Dorsal bud forms most of head, body and tail of pancreas. Ventral bud forms posterior and inferior part of the head.

Ans.2
B
Head is at the level of L2, body is at the level of L1 and tail is at the level of T12.
Anatomical continuity is through peritoneal reflection from transverse mesocolon, small intestinal mesentery, lienorenal and splenocolic ligament. Venous drainage is through superior mesenteric vein.

Ans.3
D
Mumps, ERCP, and choledochal cyst are all causes of pancreatitis.

Ans.4
A
Serum amylase is nonspecific, as it also increases in intestinal perforation, intestinal obstruction, and acute cholecystitis. ERCP is rarely indicated but is helpful in relapsing pancreatitis associated with pancreaticobiliary malunion.

Ans.5
D
Meperidine is better than morphine because the latter produces spasms of the ampulla of Vater. TPN is part of the treatment and helpful. Glucagon, somatostatin and anticholinergics are all part of the treatment. Surgical intervention is required when diagnosis is uncertain, when there are complications like pseudocyst or abscess or when the cause is surgically correctable pancreaticobiliary disease.

Ans.6
A
Chronic relapsing pancreatitis is characterised by recurrent episodes of upper abdominal pain.

Ans.7
C
Pseudo-pancreatic cyst does not have epithelial lining. Cyst lies mostly in lesser sac, surrounded by fibrous capsule, formed by stomach, duodenum, small intestine, colon and omentum.

Ans.8
D
Medical management is supportive therapy, which is generally required for 6 weeks if no improvement surgical therapy is required.

Ans.9
C
Diazoxide helps by inhibiting glucose stimulated insulin secretion. Mesoxalyl urea is the beta cell cytotoxic agent. In surgery, 95 percent resection of the pancreas is required, leaving a rim of tissue on duodenum and bile duct.

Ans.10
A
Rise in white cell count is a feature of Ranson criteria on admission, not during first 48 hours.

PORTAL HYPERTENSION

Ans.11
C
In end-to-side portocaval shunt, end of portal vein and side of inferior vena cava are anastomosed.

BILIARY ATRESIA

Ans.12
A
Type III atresia at portahepatis is the most common, about 88 percent.

Ans.13
E
A, B, C, and D are all true. In addition to these other theories indicates that loss of blood supply, abnormal bile acid, metabolism and pancreaticobiliary maljunction.

Ans.14
C
Earlier the presentation, better the prognosis. Abdominal pain, abdominal mass, and jaundice are the triad seen in choledochal cyst. Jaundice, clay-colour stool, and hepatomegaly are the triad seen in biliary atresia. Child may presents with hepatic decompensation, oesophagal variceal bleeding and infection.

Ans.15
C
Upper GIT contrast study is generally not required.

Ans.16
B
Modification by prolonging the loop of Roux-en-Y reduces the incidence of cholangitis.

Ans.17
D
All of the above.

Ans.18
E
A, B, C and D all statements are true.

Ans.19
E
Differential diagnosis also includes neonatal hepatitis, acquired obstruction like external pressure or stone, glycogen storage disease, lysosomal storage disease, G6PD deficiency and hemolytic disease.

Ans.20
C
20 cm loop is too short; about 40 cm loop of jejunum is used.

Ans.21
A
Hepatic fibrosis may increases even after achievement of good biliary drainage in 70 percent of cases. After portoenterostomy, early cholangitis is noted in 3–60 percent of cases. Portal hypertension has been seen in about 68 percent of cases. Post-surgical 5-year survival is 32 percent, and with liver transplantation about 70 percent. The relationship between time at which portoenterostomy is performed and restoration of bile flow is less than 10 weeks 65 per cent and more than 10 weeks 25 percent.

Ans.22
A
Most patients require liver transplantation within 6 months.

Ans.23
B
Triangular cord sign.

CHOLEDOCHAL CYST

Ans.24
E
There are 5 types. Type I consists of a cystic dilation of the common bile duct with normal size right and left hepatic ducts and a normal gallbladder entering the cyst. This is the most common type, making up 85–95 percent of the cases. Type II cysts are diverticular outpouchings from the common bile

duct. Type III cysts are choledochocele, dilations of the distal common bile duct located either in the duodenal wall or the head of the pancreas. Type IV choledochal cysts are similar in appearance to the extrahepatic ducts of the type I choledochal cysts with the addition of intrahepatic biliary duct dilation. Type V choledochal cysts or Caroli's disease, consists of a normal extrahepatic biliary duct system with dilated intrahepatic bile ducts.

Ans.25
D
All of the above are true.

Ans.26
C
Adult form occurs in children older than two years. The classical triad is abdominal pain, palpable mass, and jaundice. Infantile form occurs in 1–3 months of age, characterized by jaundice, acholic stool and hepatomegaly. Serum conjugated bilirubin is high. Pre-operative liver biopsy is indicated to exclude cirrhosis and malignancy.

Ans.27
C
Type I is the commonest variety, so for cyst excision with Roux-en-Y, hepaticojejunostomy is the commonest procedure. Residual cyst can develop malignant changes.

Ans.28
A
Pancreatitis is more common after choledochocele (type III) surgery. For choledochocele surgery, a longitudinal duodenal incision required to expose the intraduodenal choledochocele.

Unroofing of cyst and mucosa is re-approximated. Bile duct and pancreatic duct must be identified and calibrated. If opening is narrow, sphincteroplasty should be done. Rarely cyst located in the head of pancreas that are not amenable to internal drainage into the duodenum. For that, pancreaticoduodenectomy may be required.

Ans.29
E
The histological type adenocarcinoma can occur.

SPLENECTOMY

Ans.30
C
Squeeze spleen gently to return as much blood as possible before clamping vessels. Hemostasis during splenectomy after trauma is achieved using electrocoagulation, argon beam coagulation, plagete in suture and absorbable mash. Midline incision is preferred in splenectomy after trauma, while subcostal incision is good for elective splenectomy. It is preferable to clamp splenic artery first. Absorbable suture is used for closure of posterior peritoneum and fascia.

Ans.31
A
The incidence of infection after splenectomy in children under 16 years old is 4.4 percent, with a mortality rate of 2.2 percent. (Ref: *PubMed* -Br J Surg. 1991 Sep; 78(9):1031–8.)

HIRSCHSPRUNG'S DISEASE

Ans.32
C
Failure of migration of neural crest cells because there is deficiency of glycoprotein (e.g., fibronectin, laminin and hyaluronic acid), which guides the migration. Increase expression of class II antigen in mucosa and submucosa of patients with Hirschsprung's disease, which demonstrates possibility of immunological response against neuroblast. Mutation at long arm of chromosome number 10, causes deficient nitrous oxide synthetase. Nitrous oxide is major inhibitory mediator. Its deficiency leads to spastic condition.

Ans.33
A
In Hirschsprung's disease, there is nascence of ganglionic cells. Ganglionic cells cause contraction and relaxation of smooth muscles. Relaxation is predominant in normal condition. Increased extrinsic innervation is seen in Hirschsprung's disease. Hypertrophy of nerve bundle seen. Normally, cholinergic is excitatory and adrenergic is inhibitory, but in Hirschsprung's disease, adrenergic also becomes excitatory, leading to spastic condition of ganglionic part.

Ans.34
E
There is decreased recto-sigmoid index in Hirschsprung's disease. Addition features of Hirschsprung's disease in barium Enema are, post-evacuation radiograph, 24 hours or more shows incomplete evacuation of barium and saw tooth appearance in enterocolitis.

Ans.35
D
Hypothyroidism is one of the differential diagnoses of Hirschsprung's disease. Other differential diagnosis includes small intestinal stenosis, low imperforate anus, prematurity, meconium plug syndrome, sepsis, electrolyte imbalance, functional constipation and intestinal neuronal dysplasia.

Ans.36
D
Martin's modification is for total colonic aganglionosis.

Ans.37
E
A, B, and C are complications of surgical procedures of Hirschsprung's disease. Other complications of Hirschsprung's disease are stenosis and post-operative intestinal obstruction, post-operative enterocolitis, fecaloma, anastomotic disruption, and enterocolic fistula.

Ans.38
A
Biopsy should be taken 1–2 cm above the dentate line. Biopsy is taken from posterior wall. Rectal defect after taking biopsy should be closed by interrupted or running stitches. Stay suture helps in taking biopsy.

Ans.39
E
A, B, and C all are true statements.

Ans.40
A
It is difficult to identify transitional zone in neonates.

Ans.41
C
The specimen should be taken from posterior or lateral wall, not from anterior wall.

Ans.42
E
Hypothyroidism causes constipation.

Ans.43
C
86 per cent of patients are full term, while 14 per cent are preterm. 81 percent are boys and 19 percent are girls. Age at the diagnosis is less than one month in 43 percent of cases, one month to one year in 37 percent of cases, more than one year in 20 percent of cases. As far as clinical features are concerned abdominal distension is seen in 59 percent of cases, failure to pass meconium in 42 percent of cases, bilious vomiting in 41 percent, enterocolitis in 7 percent, perforation 3 per cent and complete bowel obstruction in 3 percent of cases. Level of disease noted as recto-sigmoid in 79 percent of cases.

Ans.44
A
Risk of future offspring is around 4 percent.

Ans.45
B
4–8 percent.

Ans.46
C
Enterocolitis is the most common late complication. Presents with abdominal distension, pain, fever and explosive watery diarrhoea. The disease may be mild or fulminant gram negative sepsis or intestinal perforation. The enterocolitis may occur prior to colostomy or after properly done pull-through.

Ans.47
C
4–5 percent.

Ans.48
E
All statements A, B, C and D are true.

Ans.49
A
10–30 percent percent of Hirschsprung's disease is associated with meconium plug syndrome.

ANORECTAL MALFORMATION

Ans.50
A
The perineal fistula needs only anoplasty.

Ans.51
B
Rectovestibular fistula.

Ans.52
D
Flat perineum is a feature of intermediate or high anorectal malformation.

Ans.53
E
All the above statements are true.

Ans.54
E
>3 cm

Ans.55
E
90 percent

Ans.56
D
Posterior segital anorectoplasty (PSARP). Colostomy is the early treatment for this condition.

Ans.57
A
This is an advantage to having long segment for mobilization at the time of definitive procedure.

Ans.58
E
Old common channel is reconstructed as neo-urethra.

Ans.59
B
A baby pushing during each bowel movement indicates that there is some feeling during defecation process and have good prognosis. Anal dilatation is started on first month. Some degree of functional disorder after repair of anorectal malformation is experienced by most of patients, due to congenital deficiencies, which are not correctable. Liquid stool, which does not distend the rectum are not felt by most of patients. Procedure in which recto-sigmoid is lost indicates reservoir is lost, leading to greater tendency to pass stool constantly.

Ans.60
D
Anocutaneous fistula is considered as low anomaly. Rectovestibular fistula is considered as intermediate/high anomaly.

Ans.61
C
Short sacrum is a feature of high anomaly.

Ans.62
C
Distal colostogram to exclude distal obstruction, shows level of rectal pouch, and also shows fistula if any.

NECROTISING ENTEROCOLITIS

Ans.63
E
All of the above are different options of management of necrotizing enterocolitis, depending upon situation.

Ans.64
A
Colon is commonest site of stricture in about 70 percent of cases.

Ans.65
A
B, C, D and E are preventive measures, in addition to breastfeeding.

Ans.66
E
Immunoglobulin administration is not a cause of NEC. Other causes include quantity and virulence of organism and deficiency in immune and non-immune system.

Ans.67
A
Metabolic acidosis is the laboratory finding, not the alkalosis in NEC.

Ans.68
C
Portal vein gas is not a feature the mesenteric vein.

Ans.69
D
Positive blood culture is not an indication for surgery. A, B, C and E are indications for surgery. Other indications include fixed dilated loop of intestine and positive paracentesis.

ANTEGRADE CONTINENT CATHETERIZABLE STOMA

Ans.70
A
It is used for antegrade enema.

Ans.71
E
Success rate is 90 percent.

Ans.72
D
In Melon's procedure prolapse of appendix least likely seen.

Ans.73
B
In wheelchair-bound patients, a higher site of stoma is usually required.

RECTAL PROLAPSE

Ans.74
D
A, B and C are precipitating factors for rectal prolapse. Other precipitating factors include rectal polyps and cystic fibrosis. Other causes of rectal prolapse include pelvic floor weakness and malnutrition.

Ans.75
E
All of the above.

Ans.76
E
Sclerotherapy is given in lateral and posterior direction. In Thiersch procedure, generally two small incisions are required, at 12 and 6 o'clock positions. Recurrence rate is 5–10 percent. Injection sclerotherapy is repeated at 4–6 weeks, if needed. Internal fixation by laparotomy, mucosal resection and anastomosis are other options of management.

Ans.77
D
One-fifth.

ULCERATIVE COLITIS

Ans.78
D
Inflammation extends proximally in contiguous manner. Ulcerative colitis is an immunological response to bacterial and chemical agent. It is an inflammatory condition of rectal and colonic mucosa. Rectum is involved in 95 percent of cases. Cobblestone appearance is a feature of Crohn's disease.

Ans.79
A
Uveitis is an extraintestinal manifestation of ulcerative colitis, not conjunctivitis.

Ans.80
D.
Loss of haustral fold is a feature of ulcerative colitis on barium enema.

Ans.81
D
Options of surgical treatment are:
1. Total proctocolectomy with permanent ileostomy
2. Kock continent ileal reservoir with nipple valve
3. Ileal pouch procedure
Distal colostomy is not an option, as it is a disease of colon and rectum. A cleaning enema is avoided before surgery because it causes acute flare-up of colitis. Indication of surgery includes persistent symptoms of ulcerative colitis, despite medical therapy, growth retardation, severe limitation of activities and unacceptable quality of life. Indication of emergency surgery is fulminant disease, which is refractory to medical therapy, extensive rectal bleeding and toxic megacolon.

Ans.82
D
Azathioprine response time is about 3 months.

CROHN'S DISEASE

Ans.83
D
Macroscopically Crohn's disease as cobblestone appearance. The entire intestinal wall increases in width. Granuloma are non-caseating. Skip lesions are common. In 50 percent of cases, both small and large intestine are involved.

Ans.84
E
Pseudo polyp is a feature of ulcerative colitis. The string sign is caused by incomplete filling of the intestinal lumen, which results from irritability and spasm associated with severe

ulceration. In such cases, the string sign is most frequently seen at the terminal ileum.

Ans.85
B
Toxic megacolon develops in ulcerative colitis.

Ans.86
D
Fistula formation is the most common complication in Crohn's disease. Fistula may develop between small intestinal loops, between small intestine and large intestine, between intestine and urinary bladder, and between intestine and skin.

Ans.87
A
Recurrence of Crohn's disease after resection is common.

Ans.88
B
The presence of perianal abscess and the fistula is often the first sign of Crohn's disease. Stoma should be avoided because of high incidence of peristomal complications.

Section 3

ABDOMEN C

INGUINAL HERNIA

Ans.1
B
Left-sided hernia in girls under two years of age is an indication of contralateral exploration, not the right sided hernia.

Ans.2
D
It is called Litter's hernia when Meckel's is the content. Irreducible hernia is called incarcerated hernia. Hernia with features of obstruction is called obstructed hernia. Hernia with compromised blood supply is called strangulated hernia. Hernia with double loops of bowel is called Maydl's hernia, and when a portion of bowel is strangulated, it is called Richter's hernia.

Ans.3
D
Failure of ligation of sac at internal ring is the cause of recurrence.

Ans.4
E
About 21 percent of hernia sac contains salpinx.

Ans.5
E
Transillumination is not definitive because thin walled infants intestine may be transilluminated as nearly as hydrocele sac. The criteria for post-operative in hospital monitoring is the

infant's post-conceptual age (gestational age + age in weeks). After 45–50 weeks of postconceptual age, the probability of life-threatening apnea is minimal; thus, infants with postconceptual age of 55 do not require in-hospital monitoring.

UMBILICAL HERNIA

Ans.6
E
All statements A, B and C are true.

Ans.7
E
80 percent

Ans.8
C
Umbilical hernia was classified as small if fascial defect is less than 0.5 cm, medium if fascial defect is 0.5–1.5 cm, and large if fascial defect is greater than 1.5 cm.

CIRCUMCISION

Ans.9
A
In the world, the commonest reason for circumcision is religious. All Muslims and Jews gets circumcised. Some part of world, especially Africa, circumcision is also done for social and cultural reasons. In the developed world, one of the common reasons is phimosis.

Ans.10
B
Meatal stenosis is one of the complication, not the dilatation.

BLEEDING PER RECTUM

Ans.11
B
Intussusception is common in infants. Common causes of bleeding per rectum in neonate are swallowed maternal blood, haemorrhagic disease of newborns, and anal fissure. Other causes in neonates include necrotising enterocolitis, malrotation, and volvulus. Common causes of bleeding per rectum in infants are anal fissures, intussusception, internal volvulus, duplication, and gastroenteritis. In toddlers and preschool children's, common causes of bleeding per rectum are anal fissure, rectal prolapse, gastroenteritis, Meckel's diverticulum, juvenile polyp, and trauma. Common causes in teenagers are polypoid disease, ulcerative colitis, haemorrhoids, and Meckel's diverticulum.

Ans.12
E
If isolated juvenile polyp, it will not come in category of Peutz-Jeghers syndrome.

Ans.13
A
Familial adenomatous polyposis (FAP) is an autosomal dominant disorder. FAP is called the "spare" type, when polyps are in hundreds, and it is called the "profuse" type when polyps are in the thousands.

Ans.14
E
Intracranial tumours (glioblastoma and meduloblastoma) are features of Turcot's syndrome.

Ans.15
A
The polyp of Peutz–Jeghers syndrome most commonly occurs in the small intestine (55 percent) but are also found in stomach, duodenum (30 per cent), and colon/rectum (15 percent).

Ans.16
C
2–6 percent of cases.

Ans.17
C
Explanation. Older children are more likely to have pathological lead point.

SHORT-BOWEL SYNDROME

Ans.18
D
Mid-gut volvulus, not the sigmoid volvulus, is the cause of short-bowel syndrome. Other causes include Hirschsprung's disease and in older children, Crohn's disease, trauma, tumour, vascular accident and surgical injuries.

Ans.19
A
Diarrhoea, not constipation, is caused by short-bowel syndrome.

Ans.20
E
There is decreased secretion of somatostatin in short-bowel syndrome. Somatostatin reduces secretion and motility.

Ans.21
C
Increased carbohydrates leads to lactic acidosis and should be avoided. Parenteral nutrition with high dose of taurine reduces the liver disease. Sulphonamide is used in eosinophilic colitis, which is one of the complications of short-bowel syndrome.

Ans.22
A
The purpose is to prolong the intestinal transit.

Ans.23
E
In general, patients with 10 cm of healthy small bowel and intact ileocecal valve have significant potential for adaptation. Adaptation to full enteral feeding occurs in about 2 years. Twenty percent do not develop progressive adaptation. Long-term survival is 80–94 percent.

MESENTERIC AND OMENTAL CYST

Ans.24
D
Mesenteric or omental cysts contain cuboidal or columnar epithelium, while cystic lymphangia has endothelial lining. A, B, C and E are features of lymphangioma.

Ans.25
B
Duplication cysts have a well-defined mucosal layer, like the adjacent bowel, while the mesenteric cyst does not have one.

Ans.26
A
Intestinal obstruction is the most common complication of mesenteric cyst. Malignancy is noted in 3 percent of cases.

DUPLICATION OF GASTROINTESTINAL TRACT

Ans.27
E
All of the above (A, B, C and D) events happening can lead to formation of duplication cyst.

Ans.28
C
Duplication cysts are solitary in 90 percent of cases, multiple in 10 percent of cases. Duplication of abdominal cysts accounts for 75 percent (mostly small intestine), thoracic 20 per cent, thoraco-abdominal 4 percent, and other 1 percent. Ectopic gastric mucosa is seen in 20 percent of cases. 75 percent enteric duplication cysts do not communicate with bowel.

Ans.29
E
Tubular variety usually occurs in distal small intestine and colon.

Ans.30
B
Diaphragmatic hernia seems to be associated with thoracic duplication cysts.

Ans.31
B
Sclerotherapy is not an option of treatment. Roux-en-Y is other option of treatment. Duodenal duplication may needs Roux-en-Y if other option, like excision or partial excision with mucosal stripping, poses danger of injury to bile or pancreatic duct.

Ans.32
C
Duodenal duplication does not communicate with the intestinal lumen.

PRIMARY PERITONITIS

Ans.33
A
Primary peritonitis is an infectious process of abdominal cavity that has no intra-abdominal source.

ACUTE APPENDICITIS

Ans.34
A
Children have small omentum, so there is less chance of mass formation but more chance of perforation. Laparoscopic appendectomy is better in obese patients and is easy to do.

Incidence of bleeding noted in laparoscopic appendectomy is more than open. Laparoscopic has shorter hospital stay.

Ans.35
E
Statement A, B, C and D are true. Appendix should be removed in malrotation because of potential confusion caused by appendix in ectopic location. Appendix should not be removed in Crohn's disease because of increased chance of fistula formation. Appendix may be used in certain GIT and urological reconstruction surgery, so it should not be removed in faecal or urinary incontinent patients.

Ans.36
E
Duration of postoperative antibiotic in catarrhal appendicitis is about 48 hours. Drain placement in perforated appendix is optional. It has the advantage of draining fluid and collection. It has the disadvantage of the chance of adhesion, infection, perforation, and fistula formation. Burring of stump is also optional. Burring of stump has the advantage of less chance of adhesion formation by retained stump and less chance of recurrent appendicitis. The disadvantages of burring stump are the chance of faecal fistula formation (if caecum is friable) and confusion by filling defect on future barium enema.

Ans.37
E
80 percent.

INTESTINAL PARASITES

Ans.38
B
Roundworm (*Ascaris lumbricoides*) is the commonest worm that causes intestinal obstruction.

Ans.39
A
Vitamin A.

Ans.40
D
Dyspnea. Ascaris pneumonia (Loeffler syndrome) causes fever, cough and dyspnoea. Sputum is blood-stained and may shows larvae.

Ans.41
D
Penicillin is not useful to treat *Ascaris lumbricoides* (roundworm) infestation.

Ans.42
A
Liver is commonest site; it is involved in 75 per cent of cases, followed by lung 21 per cent.

Ans.43
E
The sensitivity of indirect haemagglutination (I.H.A) test is about 80 percent.

LIVER ABSCESS

Ans.44
C
Indirect haemagglutination test (IHA) is positive in amoebic liver abscess. Amoebic liver abscess is more common than pyogenic, right lobe is much more commonly involved, and percutaneous needle aspiration under ultrasound guidance is preferred mode of treatment. Drainage is generally required if abscess is above 5 cm.

Section 4

UROLOGY A

URINARY INCONTINENCE, ENURESIS, AND BLADDER RECONSTRUCTIVE PROCEDURES

Ans.1
E
Spinal dysraphism appears in neurogenic causes of urinary incontinence.

Ans.2
D
Spinal cord trauma comes in category of neurogenic incontinence of urine. Other causes of neurogenic incontinence include spinal cord tumour, spinal tuberculosis, acute myelitis, cerebral palsy, sacral agenesis and spinal dysraphism.

Ans.3
C
Enuresis is normal voiding at an inappropriate time, when control is expected at 4–6 years of age. Bladder completely evacuated during voiding. Incontinence of urine is different from enuresis. Incontinence of urine is a failure of voluntary control of bladder and urethral muscle activity and constant of frequent involuntary passage of urine.

Ans.4
B
Newborn bladder capacity is 60 ml.

Ans.5
E
Overactivity of sphincter mechanism throughout filling and emptying produces functional obstruction or failure to empty.

Ans.6
D.
Deficiency of antidiuretic hormones leads to primary nocturnal enuresis.

Ans.7
C
The goal is to achieve large-capacity, low-pressure bladder and to attain adequate outlet resistance to prevent incontinence.

Ans.8
C
Use of facial sling is reversible.

Ans.9
A
Absorptive acidosis is a complication of ileocystoplasty. Alkalosis occurs in gastrocystoplasty.

Ans.10
E
Deep sleep does not trigger stress incontinence.

Ans.11
E
All statements A, B, C and D are true.

UROLITHIASIS

Ans.12
C
Urinary dilution prevents stone formation.

Ans.13
D
Increased carbohydrate intake is not known to be associated with urinary stone formation.

Ans.14
D
A, B, and C are radiopaque stones. Radiolucent stones are uric acid and xanthine.

Ans.15
C
Hypercitrateurea is not associated with urolithiasis.

Ans.16
D
All of the above A, B and C.

Ans.17
A
ESWL is used for small-sized pelvic and calyceal stone.

Ans.18
B
Struvite

Ans. 19
B
Almost all metabolic stones are in the upper tract.

Ans. 20
E
ESWL is preferred mode of treatment for stones up to 1.5 cm.

Ans. 21
D
The cysteine stones are usually pink or yellow upon removal, but later they turn to greenish due to exposure to air.

VESICOURETERIC REFUX

Ans.22
A
Short intravesical tunnel is the cause of vesicoureteric reflux. Other causes includes neurogenic bladder, ureteral ectopia, ureteral duplication and functional voiding disorder.

Ans.23
C
Grade III
Grade I is partial filling of undilated ureter.
Grade II is total filling of undilated upper tract.
Grade III is dilated calyx but fornix sharp.

Grade IV is blunt fornix, but the degree of dilatation but the degree of dilatation is greater than in lower stage.
Grade V is massive hydro-nephrosis and tortuosity of ureter.

Ans.24
E
Grade V reflux is an indication. Other indication includes noncompliance with medical management.

Ans.25
A
New hiatus is not created in extravesical approach.
In extravesical approach, ureter is mobilised, detrusor is opened, ureter is left attached to only underlying bladder mucosa and the detrusor is approximated over the ureter.

Ans.26
D
5:1
Other principles of ureteric reimplantation include good ureteric blood supply and tension-free anastomosis.

Ans.27
C
The injection should be given at 6 o'clock position to ureteric orifice.

Ans.28
E
No difficulty has been seen if secondary surgery is required after STING procedure.
Incidence in normal population of vesicoureteric reflux is 1–2 percent. E. coli is the commonest organism seen in urine culture; renal scarring is noted in 30–35 percent of cases. Cessation of vesicoureteric reflux after one injection is 76.8 percent.

Ans.29
A
Grade I is partial filling of undilated ureter. Grade II is total filling of undilated upper tract. Grade III is dilated calyces but fornix is sharp. Grade IV is blunt fornix, but the degree of dilatation is greater than in lower stages. Grade V is massive hydro-nephrosis and tortuosity of the ureter.

PERTIAL NEPHRECTOMY

Ans.30
B
The renal segment to be removed is readily identified.

URETERIC DUPLICATION, ECTOPIC URETER, AND URETEROCELE

Ans.31
C
Urinary incontinence is more often seen in female because ectopic ureter often lies beneath external urethral sphincter.

Ans.32
D
If kidney function is good, ureteric reimplantation in single system or ureteropyloplasty or double-barrel reimplantation for duplex system is justified. Patient may present with epididymitis, prostatitis. By ultrasound dilated upper moiety is easy to visualise. Methylene blue test can be used to see leakage. Bladder is filled with methylene blue, and perineum should be inspected regularly to see if there is any colourless moisture in the diaper. Upper pole heminephrectomy for duplex or nephroureterectomy for single system associated with

poor function is justified. Continent urinary diversion that uses Mitrofenoff's principle is used in very rare situation, like bilateral single ectopic ureter, when all measures fail.

Ans.33
E
Statement A, B, C and D are true.

Ans.34
A
Stenotic variety is entirely contained within the bladder. In sphinteric variety, orifice is located within the internal sphincter. Most ureterocele with a single system are orthotopic, while most ureterocele with duplex system are ectopic. Cobra-head appearance is found in the intravenous urogram (IVU). Endoscopic deflation with puncture is the first choice. If vesicoureteric reflux occurs, then ureterocelectomy with reimplantation of ureter is considered.

Ans.35
E
All A, B, C and D are true. Mega ureter and prune-belly syndrome.

MEGA URETER AND PRUNE BELLY SYNDOME

Ans.36
D
Repair of lower ureter is needed in most cases. Straightening and tapering of upper ureter is needed in 25 percent of cases as a second stage, because peristaltic wave above 15 cm of tapered lower pole ureter is ineffective.

Ans.37
A
In prune belly syndrome, there is adynamic segment of ureter.

Ans.38
E
All of the above are true.

DIVERSION AND UNDIVERSION

Ans.39
E
End ureterostomy is a variety of incontinent diversion. Other incontinent diversions are vesicostomy, nephrostomy, loop ureterostomy, ileal pouch and colonic conduit.

POSTERIOR URETHRAL VALVE

Ans.40
E
Bladder neck is secondarily narrowed. Type I posterior urethral valve is most common and is obliquely oriented obstructing diaphragm. It exhibits detrusor hypertrophy. Proximal urethra is elongated and dilated.

Ans.41
A
Antenatal ultrasound shows thick-walled trabeculated bladder with or without hydroureteronephrosis. Newborn may present with thin stream, cry during micturition, retain urine, and may have palpable bladder/palpable kidney. Infants and children may also present as failure to thrive, recurrent UTI, incontinence, dribbling of urine, anaemia and hypertension.

Ans.42
A
Dilatation of posterior urethra is seen.

Ans.43
B
In unstable patients initial vesicostomy is better option than valve ablation.

Ans.44
D
All of the above. Complications of posterior urethral valve includes hydroureter, hydronephrosis, renal failure, UTI, calculi formation, inadequate growth and hypertension.

Ans.45
B
Posterior urethral valve is distal to verumontanum.

Ans.46
D
Urodynamic abnormalities are seen in about 75 percent of cases. Urine culture is positive in 78 percent of cases.

Ans.47
D
On VCUG posterior urethral valve (PUV) shows keyhole sign because of dilated proximal urethra and hypertrophied neck of bladder.

Ans.48
D.
All of the above. Because of the back pressure PUV leads to bladder diverticulum, vesicoureteric reflux, hydronephrosis and renal failure.

Ans.49
B
DMSA scan gives information of the cortical morphology of the kidneys and is useful for evaluation of cortical scarring.

Section 5

UROLOGY B

RENAL AGENESIS, DYSPLASIA AND CYSTIC DISEASE, RENAL FUSION, AND ECTOPIA

Ans.1
B
There is continuity between glomeruli and calyces. No continuity between glomeruli and calyces is seen in multicystic kidney.

Ans.2
E
Pelvic ectopic kidney is most common ectopic variety. Thoracic is rare. Lumbar and iliac ectopic kidney is same thing, fixed above the crest of ilium but below the level of L2 and L3.

Ans.3
B
In 95 percent of cases, the lower poles of the two kidneys are joined.

PELVIURETERIC JUNCTION OBSTRUCTION

Ans.4
B
High sodium and high osmolality of foetal bladder urine is a feature that may predict future renal function.

Ans.5
D
In foetus urinary diversion is indicated in bilateral dilated renal pelvis with progressive decreasing amount of amniotic fluid, which is considered a significant feature of urinary obstruction.

Ans.6
C
Metabolic acidosis is known complication rather than alkalosis.

Ans.7
A
Obstruction usually results from intrinsic defect in smooth muscle layer of PUJ.

Ans.8
D
Severe obstruction of both kidneys leads to oligohydramnios. Antenatal hydronephrosis is diagnosed as early as first trimester of pregnancy by ultrasound and is followed by ultrasound. Posterior urethral valve is the cause of antenatal hydronephrosis in male. PUJ and ureterovesical junction are important because of antenatal hydronephrosis.

EXSTROPHY BLADDER

Ans.9
A
Abnormal overdevelopment, not the underdevelopment of cloacal membrane, prevents migration of mesenchymal tissues.

Ans.10
B
Separation of symphysis pubis is the finding.

Ans.11
C
Anus is anteriorly placed.

Ans.12
D
Vagina is often stenotic.

Ans.13
E
Exomphalos is not variant of exstrophy bladder.

Ans.14
C
Continent reconstruction is recommended at four years of age.

HYPOSPADIAS

Ans.15
E
External genitalia is masculinised by testosterone. Embryonic urethra has three separate segments. Midline fusion of labioscrotal fold forms the perineal median raphe. Glanular urethra is formed by ectodermal intrusion at the tip of glans. Mesenchyme in urethral fold forms the corpus spongiosum.

Ans.16
C
Penoscrotal, scrotal and perineal are a variety of posterior hypospadias.

Ans.17
D
Peyronie's disease is the development of fibrous scar tissue inside the penis that causes curved, painful erection. It affects people 40–60 years and older.

Ans.18
D
All are different phases of hypospadias repair.

Ans.19
D
MAGPI is used for glanular hypospadias and sometimes in subcoronal hypospadias.
In Mathieu repair flap tissue are raised from proximal to meatus. In Onlay Island FLAP, urethral plate is intact. In Mustarde procedure, tunnel is made under the urethral plate. Straightening of penis is confirmed by repeated intraoperative erection.

CLOACAL EXSTROPHY

Ans.20
A
Cloacal exstrophy is caused by rupture of cloacal membrane before urorectal septum completely descended.

Ans.21
C
Karyotype male should be converted to female with cloacal exstrophy because the phallic tissues are almost always inadequate.

Ans.22
D
At birth, things that can be done include repair of omphalocele, tabularization of intestinal plate, end colostomy and bladder closure if adequate abdominal volume. At about 4 years of age, bladder neck reconstruction, ureteral preimplantation, Mitrofanoff and gastric bladder augmentation can be done.

AMBIGUOUS GENITALIA

Ans.23
E
Gonads are symmetrical. Other features include clitoral hypertrophy, urogenital sinus defect and enlarged labioscrotum.

Ans.24
D
Karyotype is 45X or 46XY.

Ans.25
C
Removal of Mullerian structures is required when child is raised as male.

Ans.26
D
When the ovarian and testicular tissues coexists in same gonad, testes are always central and ovarian tissue is polar.

Ans.27
B
21-Hydroxylase.

TESTICULAR TORSION

Ans.28
A
Intravaginal (intratunical) torsion is common. There is abnormally high investment of spermatic cord by the tunica vaginalis, which allow testes to lie horizontally and may readily twisted by leg movement and cremaster contraction. In adolescence beyond puberty, Doppler ultrasound can be used to determine bloodflow to the testes, but before puberty, when the testes are 1–2 ml of volume, such investigation is of low accuracy.

Ans. 29
E
Idiopathic scrotal oedema is one of the differential diagnosis. Other differential diagnoses include epididymitis, mumps orchitic, and torsion of testicular appendage, fat necrosis, strangulated inguinal hernia, acute hydrocele and trauma.

UNDESCENDED TESTES

Ans.30
C
Gubernaculum is attached at lower pole of testes. Processus vaginalis grows caudally into the gubernaculum. Process of descends accomplished by 35 weeks. Androgen control regression of cranial suspensory ligaments. Mullerian inhibiting substance causes enlargement of gubernaculum.

Ans.31
D
Microcephaly leads to undescended testes because of low gonadotropin production.

Ans.32
E
Intra-abdominal testes is an arrest in descent, so it is an undescended testes.

Ans.33
C
Cremesteric muscle contraction causes retraction. Stimulation of cutaneous branch of genitofemoral nerve is responsible. Retractile testes are descended testes, but careful follow-up is required because it does not always remains descended. Sometimes fixation of testes is required.

Ans.34
E
Incidence of torsion in undescended testes is 20 percent because of mobility of testes in superficial inguinal pouch.

Ans.35
B
Beta HCG has 10 percent and LHRH has 10–50 percent success rate.

Ans.36
D
Most testicular tumours in childhood occur in normal testes.

Section 6

THORACIC SURGERY

CONGENITAL DIAPHRAGMATIC HERNIA

Ans.1
B
Central tendon of diaphragm develops from septum transversum, dorsolateral part develops from the pleuroperitoneal membrane, dorsal crura develops from the oesophageal mesenter and muscular portion develops from the thoracic intercostal muscle.

Ans.2
B
Posterolaterally at junction of lumbar and costal muscle group, the fibrous lumbosacral trigon remains as small remnant of pleuroperitoneal membrane and relies on its strength of the fusion of two muscle group in the final stage of development. Delay or failure of muscle fusion leaves this area weak, perhaps predisposing to herniation.

Ans.3
D
Umbilical hernia is the commonest congenital hernia.

Ans.4
B
If the closure of the pleuroperitoneal canal has not occurred by the time of mid-gut return to abdomen during a gestational age 9–10 weeks, abdominal viscera herniate to thoracic cavity.

Ans.5
D
At birth, symptoms depend on reactive pulmonary hypertension and pulmonary hypoplasia.

Ans.6
B
Scaphoid abdomen is the feature of diaphragmatic hernia because the viscera are herniated to thorax.

Ans.7
B
Fluoroscopy helps to differentiate Bochdalek hernia from eventration of diaphragm. In eventration, diaphragm moves paradoxically with respiratory motion. With inspiration, it goes up, and with expiration it goes down.

Ans.8
A
Polyhydramnios is one of the anatomical prognostic factors.

Ans.9
C
Plication is a procedure use for eventration of diaphragm.

Ans.10
D
For right-sided eventration, thoracic approach is preferred, whether it is due to phrenic nerve injury or congenital cause. Eventration of the diaphragm is different from congenital variety as it has normal distribution of muscle and normal central tendinous area. It can be observed for a few weeks for return of function, and during operation, no portion of muscle

needs to be excised. The muscular diaphragm may ultimately regain some function, and excision may only increase risk of injury to intradiaphragmatic portion of phrenic nerve. In congenital eventration, there is muscular aplasia or atrophy, and the thinned portion of diaphragm may be excised.

Ans.11
D
75 percent

Ans.12
B
2–5 percent of cases.

Ans.13
B
Trisomy 18.

Ans.14
C
Non-inflation of lung is a long-term problem, which should be followed.

Ans.15
D
Mediastinum shifts to opposite side.

OESOPHAGEAL ATRESIA

Ans.16
D
Fundoplication is the procedure for correction of gastroesophageal reflux if medical treatment fails. Oesophageal

dilatation is for correction of oesophageal stricture. If dilatation fails in stricture may needs resection and anastomosis or oesophageal replacement. Aortopexy may be required in severe tracheomalacia.

Ans.17
E
R stands for renal anomaly. VACTERL stands for vertebral defects, anal atresia, cardiac defects, tracheoesophageal fistula, renal anomalies and limb abnormalities.

Ans.18
E
E stands for ear deformities. CHARGE is an abbreviation for Coloboma, heart defects, atresia choanae (also known as choanal atresia), growth retardation, genital abnormalities and ear abnormalities.

Ans.19
E
Choice of operation is oesophagostomy and gastrostomy when the patient is not fit.

Ans.20
B
Identify and preserve vagus nerve. Recurrent laryngeal nerve is quite high and does not come across.

Ans.21
A
Long gap oesophageal atresia is an indication of cervical oesophagostomy.

Ans.22
C
Procedure includes Left-sided approach is preferred. Incision 1 cm above and parallel to medial third of cervical. Ligate and divide external jugular vein. Retract carotid sheath with its contents (carotid artery, vagus nerve and internal jugular vein) laterally. Identify and preserve recurrent laryngeal nerve.

Ans.23
A
Tube oesophagogram is done in prone position to visualise H-type fistula.

Ans.24
B
In neonates right-sided, while in adults left-sided pneumothorax occurs because of close adherence of aorta to oesophagus on the left side in infants, which provides additional support. Oesophagoscopy offers no diagnostic advantage and may actually enlarge the perforation, making subsequent repair more difficult. Decision of treatment in oesophageal perforation depends on site of perforation, whether perforation is free or contaminated, the interval from injury to diagnosis and systemic response to injury.

Ans.25
C
Incidence of dysphagia is about 50 percent. Only about 10 percent require surgery up to 10 years of age. Leakage is seen in 10–20 percent of cases. By one thoracotomy, the incidence of scoliosis increases to 10 percent, and by second thoracotomy it increases to 20 percent.

Ans.26
B
8–12 cm.

Ans.27
B
Oesophageal atresia with distal tracheoesophageal fistula. The incidence is A ≤ 1 percent, B 86 percent, C 1 percent, D 4 percent, and E 8 percent.

Ans.28
C
Gastrointestinal anomalies are found in 24 percent of cases.

Ans.29
B
10–20 percent of cases.

Ans.30
C
2–5 percent of cases.

Ans.31
A
Right cervical incision.

Ans.32
B
6–8 percent.

AORTOPEXY

Ans.33
A
Left anterior thoracotomy is preferred for aortopexy.

OESOPHAGEAL REPLACEMENT

Ans.34
D
All A, B and C are indications for oesophageal replacement.

Ans.35
D
Right, transverse or left colon may be used.

Ans.36
A
Right thoracotomy is preferred method of oesophageal replacement with colon, as most of thoracic oesophagus is situated more towards right side than left.

CAUSTIC INGESTION

Ans.37
B
Sodium hydroxide is an alkali. Ammonium hydro-oxide comes in the category of ammonia. Sodium hypochlorite and sodium polyphosphate are detergents. Hydrochloric acid is an acid. Other alkalis include potassium hydro-oxide. All above cause caustic stricture of oesophagus.

Ans.38
A
Acid ingestion causes coagulative necrosis, while after alkali ingestion liquefactive necrosis occurs.

Ans.39
C
Fiberoptic endoscopy is indicated within 24–48 hours. In case of pharyngeal burn with stridor, early oesophagoscopy is contraindicated because of upper airway obstruction. In case of alkali ingestion, induction of vomiting is contraindicated because the alkali is mostly neutralised by gastric acid, and consequences of acid regurgitation may induce further injury.

Ans.40
E
The grading of oesophageal injury after caustic ingestion is grade 0 is normal, grade I is hypermia, grade IIa is blister and superficial ulcer, grade IIb is deep discrete or circumferential ulcer, grade IIIa is small scattered area of necrosis, grade IIIb is extensive necrosis and perforation.

Ans.41
D
Stricture longer than 5 cm has poor prognostic sign.

GASTROESOPHAGEAL REFLUX

Ans.42
C
Gastric contraction is involve in opening mechanism of gastric junction and leads to reflux. Other factor in closing mechanism is intraabdominal length of oesophagus.

Ans.43

B

Intraabdominal length of more than 2 cm is sufficient to prevent reflux in infants. Lower oesophageal sphincter has two parts (pars abdominalis and pars thoracalis). Pars abdominalis is cornerstone for antireflux barrier. In newborns, pars abdominalis is 0.2 cm and pars thoracalis is 0.6 cm. At three months, both are 1.5 cm. This indicates rapid growth of pars abdominalis with good antireflux mechanism.

Ans.44

D

Gastroesophageal reflux changes squamous epithelium of lower oesophagus to columnar epithelium, which is called Barrett's syndrome, which may leads to adenocarcinoma.

Ans.45

C

In gastroesophageal reflux, the following investigations are helpful.
1. Barium upper GIT study, which demonstrates reflux and gastric outlet obstruction.
2. PH monitoring. Prolonged pH monitoring is the gold standard in diagnosing gastroesophageal reflux, with 95 percent sensitivity and specificity. Two parameters of pH monitoring correlate with the probability of oesophagitis, the number of episodes that exceeds five minutes and the total percentage of time that the pH is under 4.
3. Gastroesophageal scintigraphy. It is helpful because of high sensitivity and low dose of radiation. It demonstrates

gastroesophageal reflux, pulmonary aspiration and rate of gastric emptying.
4. Oesophageal manometry. It demonstrates impaired peristalsis and lower oesophageal hypotension. It has a role in motility dysfunction.
5. Maximum gastric outlet after Pentagastrin stimulation. Normal is below 5 meq/hour/10 kg. If high, it is a possible indication of surgery.
6. Bernstein test. Oesophagus is alternatively perfused with 0.1N Hcl and saline solution through nasogastric tube to evaluate signs of chest pain and irritability.
7. Endoscopy has a role in diagnosing oesophagitis, oesophageal stricture, Barrett's oesophagus and taking biopsy.

Ans.46
A
Semi-seated position (45–50 degree) is advised 24 hours a day. In addition to above thickened, frequent and small food advised.

Ans.47
D
Failure to thrive is an indication for surgery.

Ans.48
D
In Thal-Ashcraft procedure, there is achievement of intraabdominal length, fixation of intraabdominal oesophagus in place, restoration of angle of His, narrowing of oesophageal hiatus, and partial 180-degree wrap of fundus of stomach with intraabdominal oesophagus. In Nissan fundoplication, there is 360-degree complete wrap of fundus of stomach, with intraabdominal oesophagus and gastroesophageal junction.

Opening or unfolding of fundus of stomach is part of Boix-Ochoa procedure.

THORACIC CAVITY

Ans.49
B
Child with inadequate pulmonary reserve is not candidate for resection.

Ans.50
E
Actinomycosis is treated with pencilling or sulphonamide + trimethoprim.

Ans.51
C
Bronchiectasis is an abnormal dilatation of bronchi and bronchioles. Pneumonia and pertussis are the common causes. X-rays shows increased bronchovascular markings. It mostly occurs at the basal segment of lower lobe of lung. Pulmonary resection is rarely required.

Ans.52
D
Pneumonia.

Ans.53
D
Leakage in lower part causes right-sided effusion and leakage in upper part causes left-sided effusion.

Ans.54
D
Metastatic disease is much more common than primary tumour.

Ans.55
D
All mentioned tumours are frequently considered for pulmonary metastasectomy. Note: Metastasis should not be considered for resection until primary tumour is eradicated without evidence of recurrence and other sited of metastatic disease are ruled out.

Ans.56
C
Time is not a limiting factor in rigid bronchoscopy, as it is during flexible bronchoscopy because of the ability to ventilate through the sheath. The complication includes hypoxia, hypercapnia, bradycardia, laryngospasm, pneumothorax, airway oedema, bleeding and nosocomial infection. Relative contraindication includes pulmonary hypertension, bleeding diathesis, haemodynamic instability arrhythmia and hypoxemia.

Ans.57
B
Complete excision of bronchogenic cyst and duplication cyst is possible by thoracoscopy.

Ans.58
D
Pulmonary sequestration is the malformation of lung receiving blood supply from one or more aberrant systemic anomalous arteries, not the bronchogenic cyst.

Ans.59
A
Pulmonary sequestration has no bronchial comunication. Intralober is more common than extralober. Both are more common on the left side. Intralober are more common in posterior basal segment. Extralober are multiple in 40 percent of cases.

Ans.60
B
Communication with lower oesophagus is commonest. Communication is 4 percent with upper oesophagus, 11 percent with middle oesophagus, 67 percent with lower oesophagus, and 15 percent in stomach.

Ans.61
A
Cystic hygroma arises from any part of mediastinum. Other lesions that arise from any part of mediastinum include haemangioma, lymphangia and congenital aneurysm of pulmonary artery. From anterior mediastinum, teratoma and thymoma develop. From middle mediastinum, bronchogenic and oesophageal duplication cyst develop. From posterior mediastinum, neuroblastoma and ganglioblastoma develop.

Ans.62
C
Mediastinum is shifted on opposite side because of hyperinflation.

Ans.63
A
It shows delayed uptake and delayed washout of isotopes from air spaces and little blood flow from emphysematous lobe.

Ans.64
C
When cystic adenomatoid malformation compresses the oesophagus in foetus, polyhydramnios develops.

Ans.65
B
Exudative. Empyema is defined as pus (an exudate) in the pleural space. Presence of transudate is not an empyema. Fibrinopurulent is the second and organising is the third phase of empyema.

Ans.66
D
4:1

Ans.67
C
10 percent.

Ans.68
C
Upper and middle lobe is commonly involved. It rarely involve the lower lobe. There is no deficit in lung volume after the operation. Actual lung volume measured at 90 percent to 100 percent of the predicted volume with perfusion equally distributed between operated and non-operated lung.

A.69
E
In type III cystic adenomatoid malformation the entire lobe is infiltrated with bronchiole-like structure usually smaller than 0.5 cm in diameter.

Ans.70
E
Venous drainage is usually to systemic vein (Azygous vein).

Ans.71
B
Chyle shows high white cell count, predominantly lymphocytes.

CHEST WALL

Ans.72
A
Polythelia is a supernumery nipple. Polymastia is referred to as accessory breast.

Ans.73
A
Pectus excavatum is posterior depression of sternum and lower costal cartilage.

Ans.74
E
Absence of latissimus dorsi muscle is not a feature of Poland syndrome. Absence of pectoralis major or minor muscle is a feature of Poland syndrome.

Ans.75
C
Marfan syndrome occurs infrequently, less than 1 per cent of patients.

Section 7

HEAD AND NECK AND SOFT TISSUES

HEAD AND NECK

Ans.1
C
It presents as swelling in upper part of anterior triangle of neck.

Ans.2
E
All statements A, B, C and D are true.

Ans.3
E
Cleft palate is usually repaired in 6–18 months. In Pierre Robin sequence, repair should be delayed because of airway obstruction. Development of primary palate (prepalate) is related to structures anterior to incisive foramen (i.e., the face, lips, premaxilla and upper four incisor teeth). Secondary palate is related to structures posterior to incisive foramen (i.e., hard palate, soft palate and maxillary teeth). Primary palate develops during fourth to seventh week of gestation and secondary palate during sixth to seventh week. Frequency of cleft palate in general population is 0.02 percent.

Ans.4
D
Turbinate undergoes hypertrophy.

Ans.5
D
Millard's procedure is a rotational (medial) and advancement (lateral) procedure, in which cupid bow is preserved.

Ans.6
A
In solilithiasis, submandibular gland is involved in 90 percent of cases, 90 percent of which are radio-opaque. In parotid tumours 32 percent endothelial tumours (haemangioma and lymphangioma), 40 percent are benign epithelial tumours (32 percent are benign pleomorphic adenoma), and 27 percent are malignant epithelial tumours.

Ans.7
B
Cranial cleft is characterised by orbital hypertelorism (increased infraorbital distance).

Ans.8
A
Scaphocephaly is premature closure of sagittal sutures.

Ans.9
D
In Crouzon syndrome, normal intelligence is seen.

Ans.10
C
Vertical incision is made in the trachea through second, third and fourth tracheal ring.

Ans.11
D
Pyloric stenosis is not cause of torticollis. Sandifer syndrome is a combination of gastroesophageal reflux with spastic torticollis and dystonic body movements. It is a hypothesis that the positioning of head provides relief from abnormal discomfort caused by acid reflux.

Ans.12
D
Unilateral facial hypoplasia is seen by progressive asymmetry by unilateral immobilisation of face.

Ans.13
A
Indication of surgery is persistent sternocleidomastoid tightening, limiting head rotation beyond 12–15 months of age. Other indication is progressive faecal hypoplasia and presentation in children older than one year of age.

Ans.14
B
Ninety percent of branchial anomalies are second type.

Ans.15
E
Thyroglossal cyst is not derivative of second branchial arch. It is formed from persistence of thyroglossal duct. In other words, this anomaly is caused by a tract of thyroid tissue along the pathway of the embryological migration of the thyroid gland from the base of the tongue to neck.

Ans.16
C
Most are well differentiated papillary carcinoma. Solitary thyroid nodule is rare in children. When present they are most likely malignant. Cancer most frequently occurs at 15–19 years of age. Girls are affected more than boys.

SOFT TISSUE LESIONS

Ans.17
C
An imbalance in the relative cellular composition of tissue may lead to significant cellular malformation without alteration in global mass. In congenital giant hairy nevus, the melanocyte related nevus cells develops excessively in dermis. Other example is cutaneous port wine lesion, which results from excessive developmental accumulation of abnormal microvascular tissues in the dermis. Examples of malpositioning of otherwise normal structure are dextrocardia, meningocele and diaphragmatic hernia. The absence of regional absence of normal tissue is Amalia.

Ans.18
C
Syndactyly is a failure of differentiation. It is common between middle and ring finger. Syndromic features of syndactyly include Apert syndrome, Crouzon syndrome, trisomy 13, Pfeiffer syndrome, Golz syndrome and Poland syndrome. An example of transverse arrest in the development is Amalia. Examples of longitudinal deficiencies include radial club hand and ulnar ray deficiencies.

Ans.19
B
In polydactyly, most common is little finger duplication and second most common is thumb duplication. Central digit duplication is uncommon.

Ans.20
C
Conjoint twins result when inner cell mass incompletely divides after first seven days when monozygotic twining occurs. Conjoint twin with fused organs therefore usually have incomplete development, as manifested as in conjoint heart, liver, GIT and genitourinary tract. Complete division of zygote in first seven days of gestation yields monozygotic identical twins. They are identical in sex, karyotype and that they share amnion and yolk sac. Dizygotic twins result from fertilization of two separate ova and each foetus has its own amnion, yolk sac and umbilical cord. These twins may be of same or opposite sex and have different karyotype.

Ans.21
A
Thoracopagus is commonest variety of conjoint twin, constitutes 74 per cent. Other incidence: omphalopagus 1 percent, pyopagus 17 percent, ischiopagus 6 percent, and craniopagus 2 percent.

Ans.22
D
Organs potentially involved in Ischiopagus includes pelvis, intestine, genitourinary tract and liver.

Section 8

ORTHOPAEDIC

DIGITAL MALFORMATION

Ans.1
A
Syndactyly develops by failure of programmed cell death in-between digits. Superdigit is a form of syndactyly in which digit merges completely at either the proximal or distal end but are more or less separated at the other end.

Ans.2
C
Six months is a good age for surgery for syndactyly, if child is fit.

SPINA BIFIDA

Ans.3
C
Meningocele represents failure of fusion of neural folds, leaving a vertebral arch open and the unfused spinal cord or neural placodes either exposed or covered by the thin membrane. Spina bifida occulta neural deficit may or may not present at birth and may present at any age but often at 4 years of age. Spina bifida has visible lesion on surface. In lipomeningocele, there is an extension of fat in the spinal canal. Meningocele is only spinal filled fluid sac with meningeal or cutaneous covering, containing no spinal element but occasionally contains some nerve roots.

Ans.4
B
Meningomylocele is associated with hydrocephalus not microcephaly.

Ans.5
E
Chiari II malformation develops features of lower cranial nerve paresis.

TELIPES EQUINOVARUS

Ans.6
B
It shows medial deviation (concave medial border of foot).

Ans.7
E
The intrinsic causes of talipes equinovarus include neuromuscular diseases such as spina bifida, genetic diseases such as diastrophic dysplasia and whistling face syndrome.

Ans.8
B
Talus is smaller than normal. In severe cases, flexor digitorum longus and flexor halluces longus are contracted.

Ans.9
C
Surgery, if required, is indicated at 5 month of age (age close to walking).

Ans.10
B
Injury to common peroneal nerve is not a complication of surgery for telipes equinovarus.

DEVELOPMENTAL DYSPLASIA OF HIP

Ans.11
A
Hormonally mediated ligamentous laxity by oestrogen and relaxin is one of the cause of DDH.

Ans.12
D
Clunking sensation is felt during Ortoloni manoeuvre. In Ortoloni manoeuvre, femurs are abducted while lifting the hips towards socket. Barlow test shows a hip that is reducible but dislocatable, the Ortoloni test show a hip that is reduced but dislocatable, and the Ortoloni test shows that a hip that is dislocated but reducible.

Ans.13
A
DDH shows excessive lordosis.

Ans.14
B
Ultrasound is useful up to age one. After one year as femoral nucleus mature, visualization of acetabulum impaired on ultrasound. Barlow and Ortolani test has no significant role in diagnosis after 3 months, as there is more stabilised dislocation and restricted abduction.

Ans.15
B
There is hypertrophy of acetabulum labrum, which obstructs the superior boundary of acetabulum.

Ans.16
C
Anterior approach is the most commonly used method because it is more extensile, provides excellent exposure, is appropriate at any age, and is the preferred method in older children in whom the femoral head migrates far proximally and soft tissue deformity is more established. It is always required when the labrum is the major obstacle to reduce.

SEPTIC ARTHRITIS

Ans.17
D
Staph aureus is the commonest organism involved in septic arthritis. H-influenza is seen in 25 percent cases.

OSTEOMYELITIS

Ans.18
C
When infection is locally confined but not eradicated, it is called Brodie's abscess. Staph aureus is the commonest organism involved. Salmonella is the commonest organism involved in sickle cell disease. Necrotic bone is called sequestrum, and new bone formed around dead bone is called involucrum.

Ans.19
C
The first change that appears on X-rays is decreased in bone density.

FEMUR FRACTURE

Ans.20
E
In early Spica cast immobilisation for femoral fracture, there is a short hospital stay.

Ans.21
C
Skeletal traction can be applied for longer duration.

Ans.22
B
Wound care is easy in compound fracture if external fixator is used.

Ans.23
B
There is increased chance of infection by using internal fixator.

Ans.24
A
Pseudoarthrosis is late complication of femur fracture.

Ans.25
A
Compartment syndrome is an early complication in fracture femur, especially in crushed limb.

INGROWN TOENAIL

Ans.26
E
All of A, B, C and D are true causes of ingrown toenail.
1. Ill-fitting footwear. Main cause is too narrow or too short shoes, causing the nail to curl and dig into the skin.
2. Bad nail care. It includes cutting the nail too short, rounding off at or peeling off at the edges, instead of cutting straight across
3. Other factors: tight stockings, hyperhidrosis, soft tissue abnormality of toes, trauma to nail plate or toe, nail deformities, genetic susceptibility, bacterial infection and weight bearing.
4. Special condition e.g diabetes and immunosuppressive drugssuch as cyclosporine.

Ans.27
D
Statement A, B and C are true.

Ans.28
B
Operation is contraindicated when there are physical signs of ischaemia. Ankle brachial pressure index below 0.5 or toe pressure below 40 mm Hg.

Ans.29
E
Phenol ablation of nail matrix at the site of resection reduces the recurrence rate.

Section 9

TRAUMA

ABDOMINAL TRAUMA

Ans.1
E
Presence of lipase is not a criteria for labelling positive peritoneal lavage.

Ans.2
A
Stab wound needs local wound exploration.

Ans.3
C
There is no indication of magnesium administration after four blood transfusions until it is low.

Ans.4
A
Transabdominal approach is usually selected in acute cases to permit assessment of possible intraabdominal injury. However, in late cases, when adhesion may be present, a thoracic incision is preferable.

Ans.5
E
Stamm gastrostomy is constructed if extensive contamination has occurred or other injuries are present.

Ans.6
D
Fixed portion of intestine is more prone to perforation. Perforation mostly occurs on antimesenteric border. CT scan shows peritoneal fluid in the absence of solid organ injury and intestinal wall enhancement. Best repair is by simple closure or segmental resection with end-to-end anastomosis if the injury is extensive. In rare situations, physiological instability may necessitate exteriorization.

Ans.7
C
Decision of laparotomy based on physical condition, not the extent of injury as shown on CT.
Different selenography techniques include:
1. Vertical mattress sutures
2. Horizontal mattress sutures using Teflon pledgets to prevent tearing
3. Figure of eight sutures
5. Simple interrupted sutures with omental incorporation
6. Long-interrupted sutures
7. Chromic ladder sling to appropriate parenchyma, without insertion of needle

Ans.8
C
Third organism against which vaccination required is with pneumococcus not streptococcus.

Ans.9
B
Blunt trauma is more common cause than penetrating trauma. Compression occurs against vertebral column. Pancreas and

duodenum are retroperitoneal structures so relatively protected. X-rays shows air around right kidney. Serum amylase and lipase levels are high. Positive peritoneal lavage for bile and amylase is nonspecific for pancreaticoduodenal injury, as it is also positive in other intestinal perforations.

Ans.10
C
Pseudopancreatic cysts manifest within 3–4 weeks of injury. Pseudocyst is a consequence of inflammatory process or direct trauma to duct system. Treatment is medical in first 3–6 weeks. Most of these persists and not resolved spontaneously and requires drainage.

Ans.11
E
All mentioned statements A, B, C and D are true.

Ans.12
D
Penrose drain, not the radivac drain, is used for drainage of bile or blood if intrahepatic ligation is not entirely effective.

Ans.13
C
Embolization is the treatment of haemobilia if arteriogram shows aneurysm.

Ans.14
D
Grade IV hepatic injury is labelled when laceration is more than 10 cm deep. Grade I is less than 1 cm deep, grade II is 1–3 cm deep, grade III is 3–10 cm deep, grade IV more than 10 cm

deep laceration and grade V is bi-lobar tissue maceration and devascularisation.

Ans.15
E
All of the above statements are true.

UROGENITAL INJURY

Ans.16
B
Blunt trauma with disruption of bony pelvis accounts for most of posterior urethral injuries. Straddle injuries are an important cause of anterior urethral injury. Blood at urethral meatus is a very common finding. Grades of urethral injury are contusion (grade I), stretch injury (grade II), partial disruption (grade III) and complete disruption (grade IV).

Ans.17
C
Complex urethral injury is managed by suprapubic catheter and later on urethral stricture may develop, requiring urethroplasty. Delayed primary repair realignment causes less bleeding. Delayed primary realignment is contraindicated in boys with complete disruption of bladder neck. Secondary realignment is done after 6–9 months. Secondary reconstruction has fewer incidences of impotence and incontinence.

Ans.18
D
Long-term sequel of urethral injury, urethral stricture is most common (about 50 percent), impotence about 30 percent, and incontinence is about 8 percent. Bladder neck mechanism is

important to avoid retrograde ejaculation. Impotence is caused by nerve to erigentes. Urethral stricture by direct consequence of trauma may be from delayed reconstruction of urethral injury.

Ans.19
C
Grade I: Contusion. Microscopic or gross haematuria; urological studies are normal.
Haematoma—subcapsular, non-expanding without parenchymal laceration.
Grade II: Haematoma. Nonexpanding perirenal haematoma confined to renal retroperitoneum.
Laceration—less than 1 cm parenchymal depth of renal cortex without urinary extravasation.
Grade III: Laceration. More than 1 cm parenchymal depth of renal cortex without collecting system rupture or urinary extravasation.
Grade IV: Laceration. Parenchymal laceration extending through renal cortex, medulla and collecting system.
Vascular—Main renal artery or vein injury without contained haemorrhage.
Grade V: Laceration. Completely shattered kidney.
Vascular—avulsion of renal hilum, devascularizing the kidney.

Ans.20
E
Grade IV injury is labelled when complete transection with less than 2 cm devascularisation.

Ans.21
D
Grade IV urethral injury is complete disruption with less than 2 cm urethral separation.
Grade I is contusion, grade II is stretch injury, grade III is partial disruption and grade V is complete disruption with more than 2 cm urethral separation.

BURN

Ans.22
D
In one-year-old child, head constitutes 19 percent. By advancement in medical science 50 percent of burn has about 98 percent survival. Parkland formula is 4 ml/kg/percent of burned surface area in addition to maintenance fluid. In four-year-old child, one lower limb constitutes 15 percent of body surface area. Fifty percent of Parkland formula fluid should be given in first 8 hours.

Ans.23
D
Povidone iodine is a painful application, so needs good analgesic and monitor of thyroid function. Silver sulphadiazine is a painless application. Mefenide acetate penetrates eschar while silver nitrates does not penetrate eschar. Gentamicin is a broad spectrum antibiotics.

Ans.24
C
Bacterial invasion is suspected when bacterial count is more than 107 organism/gram of tissue. Features of septicaemia include hypothermia, hyperthermia, paralytic ileus, altered mental

status, tachycardia, unexplained acidosis, thrombocytopenia, leucocytosis or hyperglycaemia.

Ans.25
E
All statements are true. Increases in catecholamine causes mesenteric vasoconstriction, which leads to decrease in mucosal integrity that in turn causes bacterial translocation resulting in necrotizing enterocolitis.

Ans.26
B
Pink wound with bulla is features of partial thickness burn. Full-thickness skin burn is usually dry.

Ans.27
A
Saponification of fat is a feature of alkali burn.

Ans.28
C
If fascial compartmental pressure is increased, do fasciotomy to save limb.

Ans.29
B
In carbon monoxide poisoning, carboxyhaemoglobin rises more than 10 percent.

Ans.30
C
40 percent.

THORACIC TRAUMA

Ans.31

A

Pulmonary contusion is potentially life-threatening, not immediately life-threatening. Other immediate life-threatening injuries include myocardial contusions, aortic disruption, ruptured diaphragm and tracheobronchial disruption. Other immediate life-threatening injuries include open pneumothorax and flail chest.

Ans.32

B

Lung contusion is the commonest thoracic injury (50 percent). Other incidences are rib fracture 30 per cent, pneumothorax 24 percent, and haemothorax 9 percent. Rare thoracic injuries include diaphragmatic rupture, aortic, bronchial, and oesophageal injuries, lung laceration, cardiac contusion and cardiac laceration.

Ans.33

C

Chest intubation is required for tension pneumothorax. Open pneumothorax with major chest wall defect needs immediate thoracotomy. Other possible indications of immediate thoracotomy include oesophageal perforation, diaphragmatic rupture, and massive or continuous air leak, indicating injury to major airway.

Ans.34
C
Hoarseness indicates direct laryngeal or tracheal injury. Tracheal deviation implies tension pneumothorax and massive haemothorax.

Ans.35
D
Reversible cardiovascular failure is one of the inclusion criteria for ECMO, not the exclusion criteria.

CHILD ABUSE

Ans.36
A
Fractures at various stages of healing are seen in battered baby syndrome. In shaken baby syndrome, the baby is shaken violently while being held by the torso, which causes acceleration and deceleration injury of the head, neck and trunk. Acute brain injury occurs, such as subdural and subarachnoid bleeding with cerebral contusion, with no external evidence of head haematoma.

BIRTH TRAUMA

Ans.37
E
Among fractures, clavicular fracture is the most common in birth injuries.

Section 10

ONCOLOGY

GENERAL ONCOLOGY

Ans.1
A
Cancers in children, from common to rare, are leukaemia, brain tumour, lymphoma, neuroblastoma, sarcoma, Wilms tumour, osteosarcoma and liver tumours.

Ans.2
C
The higher the mitotic activity, the more sensitivity to radiation. Other principles include total cumulative dose depends primarily in the type of tumour being treated not the age or weight of the child. Maximise the irradiated normal tissues to repair by use of hyperfractioned radiation therapy.

Ans.3
B
Busulfan and bleomycin cause restrictive lung disease.

CENTRAL NERVOUS TUMOURS

Ans.4
A
Astrocytoma is the commonest CNS tumour, accounting for 32 percent, craniophrangioma 5.8 per cent, meningioma 2.8 percent, mixed meningioma 3.6 percent, pinocytoma 0.5 percent, PNET 17.6 percent, ependimoma 5.7 percent, rhabdoid 12 percent, oligodandrioglioma1.9 percent, ganglioma 7.9

percent, germ cell tumour 7.9 percent, choroid plexus 2.6 percent, pituitary adenoma 1.1 percent, metastatic tumour 1.0 percent.

Ans.5
B
Infratentorial is commonest (45–60 percent).
Supratentorial hemispheric is 25–40 percent.
Supratentorial midline is 15–20 percent.
Supraseller and pineal region tumour fall into the category of supratentorial midline tumours.

Ans.6
A
MRI is better than CT. MRI provides multiplane images that are helpful in planning surgery and with new imaging sequence and spectroscopy, may even provide specific diagnosis. Intramural calcification, which is seen in craniopharyngioma and teratoma, is poorly seen with MRI. Optimal characterisation of tumour may require both CT and MRI.

Ans.7
A
Astrocytoma is usually benign.

Ans.8
E
Excision is ideal treatment for arteriovenous malformation. Clipping of feeding vessels without resection is treatment for residual malformation.

Ans.9
D
A longer duration of exposure of the tumour to a given cell cycle-specific agent might lead to greater efficacy. Recovery of normal tissues takes an average of 21 days, so after chemotherapy, an interval is required. Combination chemotherapy is better than single-agent chemotherapy, as not all the cells in the tumour are equally sensitive to chemotherapeutic agent. Maximally tolerated dose should be administered. Dose intensity can be maximised by increasing the total dose of an agent or by shortening the time interval between the doses. Maximum tolerated dose should be administered. Dose intensity can be maximised by increasing the total dose of an agent or by shortening the time interval between the doses. For a given increase in dose, a greater increase in tumour cell killing is achieved. For example, if the dose of cyclophosphamide is increased twofold, a tenfold increase in tumour cells killed can be observed. Neoadjuvant chemotherapy is given before the operation to shrink the primary tumour and make surgical resection possible or less injurious or allow reduction of radiation field size or total dose. Adjuvant chemotherapy is for no metastatic tumour after removal of the primary tumour. The goal of adjuvant chemotherapy is to eliminate disease not detectable by slandered radiographic means beyond the primary tumour site.

TERATOMA AND GERM CELL TUMOUR

Ans.10
D
Yolk sac endodermal sinus tumour develops from extraembryonic differentiation.

Ans.11
E
All statements A, B, C and D related to types of sacrococcygeal teratoma are true.

Ans.12
C
Alpha-fetoprotein does not rise in seminoma.

Ans.13
C
Beta HCG is secreted in germ cell tumour containing trophoblastic component (e.g., choriocarcinoma).

Ans.14
A
Sacrococcygeal area is the commonest site of germ cell tumour. According to site, germ cell is divided as follows.
Extragonadal
(a) Sacrococcigeal 41 percent
(b) Mediastinal 6 percent
(c) Abdominal 5 percent
(d) Intracranial 6 percent
(e) Head and neck 4 percent
(f) Vagina 1 percent
Gonadal
(a) Ovarian 29 percent
(b) Testicular 7 percent

Ans.15
B
Age greater than eleven years results in bad prognosis.

Ans.16
E
Radiation is rarely used in this condition.

Ans.17
A
Leydig cell tumour is gonadal stromal cell tumour.

Ans.18
C
Teratoma is commonest testicular tumour accounts 54 percent.

SARCOMA

Ans.19
B
It has potential to differentiate into skeletal muscle.

Ans.20
A
Head and neck is the commonest site and accounts for 35 percent of cases. Others include genitourinary without prostate and urinary bladder 16 percent, prostate and bladder 10 percent, limbs 19 percent and others 20 percent.

Ans.21
C
Commonest histological type of rhabdomyosarcoma is embryonal, which accounts for 54 percent. Others include botroid 4.5 percent, alveolar 18.5 percent, pleomorphic 0.5 percent, and undifferentiated 6.5 percent.

Ans.22
E
Botroid has the best prognosis.

Ans.23
E
None of the above.
In the clinical group classification of rhabdomyosarcoma, statement A is IIA, statement B is IIB, statement C is III, statement D is IV. Category IIC is explained as microscopic residual tumour at primary site and pathological positive lymph node.

Ans.24
E
Orbit is considered a favourable site. Other favourable sites of rhabdomyosarcoma are superficial head and neck, testes, vagina and uterus.

Ans.25
B
For the osteosarcoma of the long bones long-term survival is about 68 percent.

OVARIAN LESIONS

Ans.26
D
Peutz Jeghar syndrome is associated with granulosa cell tumour, ovarian cystadenoma and sex cord stromal tumour. Corpus luteal cysts are usually small and asymptomatic.

Ans.27
C
Granulosa cell tumour is the most common variety of sex cord stromal tumour.

Ans.28
C
Choriocarcinoma shows normal alpha-fetoprotein and high beta HCG.

LIVER TUMOURS

Ans.29
B
Hepatoblastoma is the commonest (43 percent). Hepatocellular carcinoma has 23 percent incidence, sarcoma 6 percent, mesenchymal hamartoma 6, percent and adenoma 2 percent.

Ans.30
A
The mean age children develop hepatoblastoma is 3.5 years. The hepatoblastoma is an embryonal tumour that typically develops at 1–3 years of age.

Ans.31
E
Thrombocytopenia develops from release of cytokines from tumour.

Ans.32
D
Histological subtypes of hepatoblastoma are as follows.
1. Epithelial
(a) Foetal 31 percent, (b) embryonal 19 percent, (c) macrotrabacular 05 percent, and (d) small cell 03 percent.
2. Mixed epithelial/mesenchymal
(a) Teratoid 10 percent, (b) Nonteratoid 34 percent.

Ans.33
D
Diploid tumour has somewhat better prognosis than aneuploidy tumour.

Ans.34
B
Approximately 75 percent of primary liver tumours are malignant.

WILMS TUMOUR

Ans.35
E
Bilateral renal involvement is stage IV disease. Tumour produces renin, which causes hypertension. BFGF is produced in urine and has prognostic value. WT1 and WT2 are tumour suppressor genes and must be inactivated to cause the cancer. Stage I disease is limited to kidney and renal capsule; sinus and vessels are not involved. Involvement of capsule, sinus or vessels is considered stage II disease.

Ans.36
B
5–10 percent.

Ans.37
C
75 percent.

LYMPHOMA

Ans.38
A
Discharge from lymph node is a feature of tuberculous lymphadenitis.

Ans.39
D.
Ninety per cent of these present as abdominal tumours.

Ans.40
C
Both Burkitt's and non-Burkitt's lymphoma are varieties of undifferentiated lymphoma.

Ans.41
C
Neuroblastoma develops from posterior mediastinum. Other mediastinal masses developing from posterior mediastinum include bronchogenic and enteric duplication cyst. Thymoma, teratoma, dermoid cyst and germ cell tumours develop in anterior mediastinum.

Ans.42
B
Lymphoma is most common. The incidence is like lymphoma 41 percent, neurogenic tumour 33 percent, germ cell tumour 7 percent, mesenchymal tumour 7 percent, cystic lesion (such as pericardial, bronchogenic and enteric) 7 percent, and thymic lesion 2.5 percent.

Ans.43
C
Urinary catecholamine measurement is indicated in posterior mediastinal masses.

Ans.44
E
None of the small, round cell tumours are associated with increased serum alpha-fetoprotein level.

Ans.45
D
Hepatoblastoma is not a small blue cell tumour. In addition to A, B, C and E, other blue cell tumours include neuroblastoma.

PHEOCHROMOCYTOMA

Ans.46
E.
Organ of Zuckerkandl is chromaffin body, derived from the neural crest, located at the bifurcation of the aorta or at the origin of inferior mesenteric artery.

Ans.47
A
Paediatric pheochromocytoma is less malignant 3 percent, compared to adult 10 percent.
The incidence of bilaterally in children 20–50 percent, while adult 10 percent.
Sustained hypertension in children 90 percent, while adult 50 percent.
Familial pattern in children 10 percent, while adults 3 percent.
Extra-adrenal site in children 30 percent, while adults 10 percent.

Ans.48
D
Most characteristic clinical feature of pheochromocytoma is hypertension.

Ans.49
D
About 3 percent of child hood tumours are malignant.

Ans.50
E
MIBG is a radioisotope scan for localization of pheochromocytoma.

NEUROBLASTOMA
Ans.51
C
Diarrhoea is because of VIP secretion, hypertension because of production of catecholamine, proptosis because of ocular metastasis, and bleeding because of thrombocytopenia. Horner's syndrome is when the tumour arises from upper mediastinum involving stellate ganglion.

Ans.52
B
Stage I, II and IV-S have a good prognosis, while stage III and IV have a poor prognosis. Age less than one year has a good prognosis, while more than one year has a bad prognosis. Adrenal gland and celiac axis are sites of a bad prognosis. Elevated level of serum ferritin indicates a bad prognosis. On histology stroma rich has a good prognosis, while stroma poor has a bad prognosis.

Ans.53
D
Neuroblastoma shows features of Horner's syndrome.

Ans.54
B
One of the presentations of neurogenic duplication cyst is paraplegia.

Ans.55
E
Stage IV-S

Ans.56
B
Neuroblastoma commonly causes downward displacement of kidney.

BONE TUMOURS

Ans.57
D
X-rays in osteosarcoma may demonstrate perpendicular or radiating striations, called "sunburst."

TESTICULAR TUMOUR

Ans.58
E
Most common malignant tumour is germ cell tumour.

Ans.59
B
Stage II

Ans.60
D
Alpha-fetoprotein level comes to normal after 25–30 days of surgery.

Ans.61
C
Gonadoblastoma.

Ans.62
A
Leydig cell tumour is gonadal stromal cell tumour.

Section 11

VESSELS AND LYMPHATICS

VASCULAR MALFORMATION

Ans.1
E
Arteriovenous malformation may be associated with hemi-hypertrophy of limb because of enhanced blood flow.

Ans.2
C
Compression of renal arteries or its branches leads to hypertension because of renin angiotensin mechanism.

Ans.3
B
Midaortic syndrome is associated with narrowing of aorta.

Ans.4
E
Varicose vein is not a feature of Klippel-Trenaunay syndrome.

Ans.5
A
Haemangioma is a localised condition, not a diffuse one.

Ans.6
A
Arteriovenous malformation is usually fast flow, while complex combined vascular malformation is usually slow flow.

Ans.7
E
Any of the above-mentioned sclerosing agents can be used in the management of lymphatic malformation.

Ans.8
B
Haemangioma is the most common soft-tissue tumour in infancy, not the third-most common.

Ans.9
E
Cystic hygroma is a variety of lymphatic malformation.

Ans.10
A
Most haemangioma does not require treatment, and more than 50 per cent are naturally involute.

LYMPHATIC MALFORMATION

Ans.11
D
Cervicofacial and cervicomediastinal has about 33 percent mortality.
Intrathoracic, intraabdominal, trunk and extremities have low mortality.
Mortality in general is 3.5–5.7 percent.
About 65 percent are apparent at birth and 90 percent are apparent by the end of second year of life.

Ans.12
D
Fluid in chylothorax contains more than 60 percent lymphocytes. Lymphangioma simplex is composed of small (capillary-sized) lymphatic channels, while cavernous lymphangioma comprises dilated lymphatic channels. Cystic hygroma and other variety of lymphatic malformation do not undergo malignancy. Bleomycin, OK432, serial laser therapy and surgery are all different ways of treating lymphangioma. In chylous ascites, internal drainage by percutaneous shunt is a possible treatment.

Ans.13
C
Primary lymphedema is one in which there is lymphatic aplasia. There are three primary types: congenital is at birth, praecox presents before 35 years of age and Tarda presents after 35 years of age. Secondary variety of lymphedema is caused by radiation, tumours, fibrosis, or inflammation. Primary lymphedema is more common than secondary. In Charles method, skin and subcutaneous tissues are removed down to the muscles and denuded surface is covered by split-thickness skin graft. In Homan's method of excision surgery, excision of subcutaneous tissues and deep fascia and creation of thick skin flaps, which are used to cover the excised area, rather than skin grafts.

Ans.14
C
50–70 percent appears at birth.

Ans.15
E
Parkes-Weber syndrome is a fast-flow vascular malformation.

Ans.16
E
Ulceration and bleeding is common feature to both haemangioma and vascular malformation.

Section 12

ANATOMY FOR PAEDIATRIC SURGEONS

THORAX

Ans.1
A
In the diaphragm development, the septum transversum forms central tendon, the posterolateral part is formed by pleuroperitoneal membrane and crura are formed by dorsal mesentery of oesophagus and contribution from body wall.

Ans.2
A.
This anatomy is important to know while mobilising oesophagus, fundoplication, surgery for diaphragmatic hernia and oesophageal replacement.

Ans.3
A
It originates in abdomen, leaves abdomen through aortic opening and drains in superior vena cava. The left intercostal and bronchial vein drains through the hemi-azygos vein and hemi-azygos vein drains in azygos vein. This anatomy is important to know for paediatric surgeons, especially during repair of oesophageal atresia, when the azygos vein is ligated and divided.

Ans.4
E
Both anterior and posterior gastric nerves arise from oesophageal plexus and contain both vagal and sympathetic fibres.

Ans.5
D
It has cortex and medulla. It is large at birth and atrophied before puberty. It lies in front of trachea. It is derived from third pair of pharyngeal pouches. It contains mainly lymphocytes.

Ans.6
D
Oesophageal opening is in diaphragm is at the level of tenth thoracic vertebrae.

Ans.7
A
Trachea has 15–20 incomplete hyaline cartilage rings.

Ans.8
C
The oblique and horizontal fissures divide in their upper, middle and lower lobes. Lingula is in the left lung.

Ans.9
B
Thoracic duct arises in the abdomen from cisterna chyli and enters in thorax through the aortic opening of diaphragm. This anatomy is important for the management of chylothorax.

ABDOMEN

Ans.10
C
Umbilical cord is covered by amnion and contains two umbilical arteries and left umbilical vein (the right vein is obliterated). Neither the vitellointestinal duct nor the urachus is normally patent at birth, though obliterated remnant of each may be seen. This anatomy is important for cannulation of umbilical vein, umbilical cut down and pathology of patent urachus and vitellointestinal duct.

Ans.11
C
Lateral muscles are not directly attached with rectus abdominis. The aponeurosis of internal oblique splits to enclose the rectus abdominis in the umbilical region. The sheath is reinforced anteriorly by external oblique and posteriorly by transverse abdominis. This anatomy is important to know, especially for laparotomy and appendectomy.

Ans.12
E
Posterior wall is formed by peritoneum and fascia tranversalis. They are reinforced by conjoint tendon (i.e., behind the superficial inguinal ring). This anatomy is important to know especially for herniotomy, PPV ligation and orchidopexy.

Ans.13
E
Pampiniform plexus is the network of many small veins in spermatic cord. The three fascia are (a) the internal spermatic fascia, which is the continuation of the fascia transversalis, (b)

the cremasteric fascia and muscle, which is continuous with the internal oblique muscle, and (c) the external spermatic fascia, which is continuous with external oblique muscle. The three arteries are testicular, cremaster, and artery to ductus deferens. The three nerves are the genital branch of the genitofemoral nerve, the Ileoinguinal nerve, and the sympathetic nerve. One muscle is the cremaster muscle.

Ans.14
B
Drainage is to para-aortic lymph nodes.

Ans.15
E
Kidney develops from metanephros.

Ans.16
B
The lesser omentum passes inferiorly, meets and encloses from above downward to the oesophagus, stomach and initial part of duodenum. Epiploic foramen is bounded anteriorly by the free edge of lesser omentum, superiorly by the liver, posteriorly by the inferior vena cava and inferiorly by the duodenum. The free edge contains the bile duct, hepatic artery, and portal vein. This anatomy helps to understand in the development and management of pseudo-pancreatic cyst.

Ans.17
D
Sigmoid mesocolon is attached on the posterior pelvic wall along line whose apex lies over left sacroiliac joint.

Ans.18
A
Peritoneum covers only its anterior surface. Intra-abdominal oesophagus anatomy is important to know for gastroesophageal reflux and fundoplication.

Ans.19
B
Stomach is lined completely by columnar epithelium and contains three different types of glands. The cardiac glands secrete mucus only. The acid and enzyme secreting glands are largely found in the body. The pyloric gland in the antrum produces mucus and the hormone gastrin. The above anatomy is important to know, especially for gastric replacement of the oesophagus and portal hypertension.

Ans.20
C
Most of duodenum is retroperitoneal. The ascending part of the duodenum is anterior to the portal vein, bile duct, and gastroduodenal artery. Clinical significance of this anatomy especially for Kocher manoeuvre, surgery for duodenal atresia and choledochal cyst.

Ans.21
D
The root of mesentery passes from the left side of second lumbar vertebrae to the right sacroiliac joint. It crosses from left to right, left psoas, aorta, inferior vena cava, right gonadal vessels, right ureter and right psoas muscle.

Ans.22
E
The ileocecal orifice opens on its medial side.

Ans.23
E
Its length is variable in children.
This appendicular anatomy is important to know for appendectomy, Melon's procedure and Mitrofenoff's procedure.

Ans.24
A
Its branches are gastric, common hepatic, and splenic arteries. Superior mesenteric artery arises directly from aorta. This anatomy is important to know for surgery on foregut and its derivatives (e.g. splenectomy, hepatic lobectomy, and gastric replacement of the oesophagus).

Ans.25
A
Blood supply of adrenal gland comes from superior, middle, and inferior adrenal arteries, which arises from inferior phrenic artery, abdominal aorta and renal artery respectively.

Ans.26
E
Portal vein and renal vein has no connection. This anatomy is important to know for the management of bleeding due to portal hypertension and shunt procedures.

Ans.27
C
Although largely covered by peritoneum, the two layers of coronary ligaments diverge to enclose a part of the diaphragmatic surface posteriorly, which is bare of peritoneum.

Ans.28
E
Parasympathetic fibres from both vagus supply the liver through anterior gastric nerve, while sympathetic fibres supply it from the coeliac plexus along hepatic arteries.

Ans.29
E
Bile duct enters in duodenum about 10 cm from pylorus.

Ans.30
D
Columnar epithelium lines the whole biliary tract.

Ans.31
A
Its anterior surface is directly related to a greater curvature of the stomach.

Ans.32
D
It is covered by peritoneum anteriorly and inferiorly. The main pancreatic duct joins the bile duct in the ampulla. The accessory duct draining the uncinate process may open separately into the duodenum proximal to duodenal papilla but frequently joins the main pancreatic duct.

PELVIS

Ans.33
A
Five vertebrae usually fuse and form the sacrum.

Ans.34
A
Levator ani muscle is supplied by third and fourth sacral nerves and the pudendal nerve and is under voluntary control.

Ans.35
C
The venous drainage through the superior rectal vein to the inferior mesenteric vein. There are also important anastomosis with the inferior rectal branches of the internal pudendal vein.

Ans.36
E
External sphincter is a voluntary muscle supplied by inferior rectal nerve and is reinforced by levator ani muscle.

Ans.37
B
Superior surface of bladder in both sexes is covered by peritoneum and the upper part of the posterior surface in the male.

Ans.38
E
The round ligament extends from upper lateral angle of the uterus through the broad ligament to the deep inguinal ring and then through the inguinal canal and ends in the labium magus.

It is continuous with the ovarian ligament and is the remnant of the gubernaculum of the ovary.

Ans.39
A
Lymphatic drainage is to para-aortic lymph nodes.

Ans.40
C
It does not open directly in the prostatic urethra. It joins the duct of seminal vesical and forms ejaculatory duct, which opens in the prostatic urethra.

Ans.41
E
Penis drains to superficial inguinal lymph nodes.

Ans.42
A
The posterior wall of prostatic urethra is marked by elevation, the prostatic utricle on each side of which enters an ejaculatory duct. In to the groove on each lateral side opens 20–30 prostatic ducts. This anatomy is important to know, especially during fulguration of the posterior urethral valve.

Ans.43
A
Pudendal nerve arises from sacral plexus.

Ans.44
A
Cisterna chyli leads directly in the thoracic duct which opens into the left internal jugular vein.

Ans.45
E
External sphincter is supplied by pudendal nerve S2 to S4.

UROGENITAL SYSTEM

Ans.46
E
Cloacal eminence is a single midline structure developing adjacent to midline allantois. It becomes genital tubercle, which forms clitoris in the female and the glans penis in male. The cloacal (labioscrotal) swelling forms the labia majora in the female and scrotum in male. The genital folds form the labia minora in the female and the body of penis in the male. This embryology is important to understand the pathogenesis of hypospadias, ambiguous genitalia, and other external genital anomaly.

Ans.47
C
Kidneys are surrounded by perinephric fat and enclosed by part of fascia tranversalis, which separate each of them from suprarenal gland.

Ans.48
A
The abdominal course is similar in males and females, while their course in the pelvis is different in the two sexes.

Ans.49
D
The inferior vena cava lies anterior to the right suprarenal gland.

Ans.50
E
Gonadal vessels arise directly from the aorta.

Ans.51
B
Left gonadal veins drains in the left renal vein while the right is the tributary of inferior vena cava.

LIMBS
Ans.52
D
Epiphysis contributes in the length of long bones. The increase in the girth occurs by lying down of bones by periosteum. Clinical significant damage of epiphysis leads to shortening of long bones.

Ans.53
C
The apex is bounded by superior border of scapula, outer border of first rib and middle third of clavicle.

Ans.54
E
Cords are named according to their arrangement around the middle part of axillary artery.

Ans.55
A
It is a triangular fossa.

Ans.56
D
Femoral artery forms behind mid-inguinal point (mid-way between anterior superior iliac spine and pubic symphysis).

Ans.57
C
The arrangement, from superficial to deep is tibial nerve, popliteal vein and popliteal artery.

Ans.58
D
Great saphenous vein passes anterior to the medial malleolus and enters in femoral vein in upper thigh. Venous blood flows from superficial to deep venous system.

HEAD AND NECK

Ans.59
E
Anterior fontanelle is closed by 18 months.

Ans.60
C
Lateral rectus is supplied by abducent nerve.

Ans.61
A
First lower incisor tooth erupts at six months of age.

Ans.62
A
In hard palate, the incisive foramen transmits terminal branch of greater palatine artery and nasopalatine nerve. The greater and lesser palatine nerves have their own opening in the posterolateral aspect of the palate. The palatine process develops from the maxillary process, the palate being completed anteriorly in the midline by the frontonasal process and posteriorly by horizontal process of palatine bone.

Ans.63
D
Submandibular duct opens at the base of frenulum.

Ans.64
B
Posterior border is formed by trapezius muscles.

VERTEBRAL COLUMN

Ans.65
D
There is no disc between C1 and C2.

Ans.66
A
Between the bony ligamentous wall of the canal and the dura is the fat-filled space with emerging spinal nerves and the internal vertebral venous plexus.

www.ingramcontent.com/pod-product-compliance
Lightning Source LLC
Chambersburg PA
CBHW020725180526
45163CB00001B/108